# More Natural Remedies

Phylis Austin
Agatha M. Thrash, M.D.
Calvin L. Thrash, Jr., M.D.

Thrash Publications
Seale, AL 36875

# Table of Contents

# Table of Contents

## AGORAPHOBIA

Hundreds of thousands of Americans are handicapped by a little known and less understood mental disorder called agoraphobia. It is the commonest phobia (abnormal fear) seen by psychiatrists, and is a fear of being alone or in public places. The word "agoraphobia" comes from a Greek word "agora" which means "a place of assembly" or "gathering place." The term appeared in the medical literature as early as 1891.

Most agoraphobia sufferers are women, and most develop symptoms between the ages of 15 and 35. The mean age of onset is 24 years. Symptoms include attacks of panic, tension, dizziness, sweating, nausea, depression, obsessions (preoccupations with unreasonable or irrational ideas), and depersonalization (a temporary sensation of strangeness or unrealness). The disease often occurs shortly after a major problem, accident, severe illness, or mental depression.

Onset of symptoms may be sudden. The patient may be standing in the check-out line at the local supermarket when she suddenly feels great anxiety, weakness, dizziness, and rapid heartbeat. She may report a lump in her throat. She may feel that she is unable to breathe and may take short, rapid breaths producing hyperventilation. She may be unable to move for several moments, or may flee to some location she perceives as safe. Because avoiding the specific situation that produces fear brings control of anxiety, many agoraphobics refuse to leave their homes for months, or even years at a time. This withdrawal prevents the development of coping skills, and worsens the problem.

The episode may last only a few minutes or several hours. After the acute phase the patient may feel fine, and many months may pass before the next episode. There may be a series of episodes over a period of several years before the patient begins to limit her activities. The disease runs a course of incomplete remission and relapse, and at times patients do things that they were previously too frightened to venture.

Many people are able to cover up their fears from all but the immediate family so it is difficult to ascertain the rate of incidence, but one study suggests that 63 out of 1,000 people are afflicted with it. About two-thirds of agoraphobics seen by psychiatrists are women.

Agoraphobics may feel more comfortable in the presence of a trusted friend – – human or animal – and become dependent on them. They perceive these friends as places of security during an attack. Some agoraphobics become dependent on inanimate objects.

Some are able to hold down jobs, but others are so overwhelmed by their fears that they become housebound. They are frightened of going out into open streets, stores, and crowds, but closed places such as theaters and churches also evoke panic. They fear travel on trains, buses, ships, and airplanes, but most can tolerate cars. If they do not have to anticipate the trip they may be able to perform it, but knowing in advance of a forth-coming trip may produce intense anxiety of such severity that they cannot take the trip. In an emergency such as a house fire or an accident, agoraphobics may temporarily overcome their fears, and function somewhat normally, but once the emergency is over they are again overwhelmed.

Agoraphobics are sometimes able to move about freely in the dark, in an area they could not enter in daylight. Some report that wearing dark glasses in daylight hours is helpful. Hot weather often worsens symptoms, as does fatigue. Illness exacerbates agoraphobia, particularly if the patient is confined to bed, as they lose practice in going out. This makes it more difficult to resume activities after the illness.

Some authorities on agoraphobia report that symptoms of a panic attack and those of hypoglycemia (low blood sugar) are very similar. Dr. Alan Goldstein, director of the Temple University Medical School Agoraphobia and Anxiety Center has observed that agoraphobics often eat lots of sweets. Eliminating sweets and caffeine, which is known to induce symptoms of anxiety, will be quite helpful in patients with any type of anxiety. Dr. Philip Bate of the Maitland, Florida Psychological Clinic feels that white flour as well as sugar must be eliminated.

Researchers at Boston University report that they have cured some cases of agoraphobia by teaching the patients to breathe properly. Women who wear tight-fitted clothing become chest-breathers, unable to take a deep inspiration. Gases in the lungs are not fully exchanged which produces a stress on the body. When anxiety begins to build these people breathe faster, in shallow breaths. Carbon dioxide is blown off too rapidly, creating a sensation of air hunger. The decreased carbon dioxide tension stimulates respiration and they begin breathing still faster, producing the fast heart rate typical of agoraphobic attacks. Clothing should be loose enough that they can breathe with the diaphragm which permits adequate air exchange.

Thought-stopping has been used with a number of phobias. The patient should select a pleasant, relaxing scene or subject, and when anxiety begins to build the patient says to herself "Stop." She may find it necessary to shout "STOP!" aloud at the beginning of the program, but as time goes on she will be able to make the word a mental command. At the stop command the patient should switch her thoughts from the anxiety to the previously selected subject. One group of patients reported reduction of fearful thoughts by following this procedure for four weeks; as time progressed they had fewer and fewer anxiety-producing thoughts.

Some cases of agoraphobia are being successfully treated with desensitization therapy. The patient, in a completely relaxed state, imagines the anxiety-producing scene. Because anxiety and relaxation are incompatible the anxiety decreases as the patient learns to substitute relaxation for it. The patient begins by imagining situations that produce only minor stress and gradually works up to the most stressful. If the agoraphobic takes a deep breath, releases it slowly while consciously relaxing, and accepts the panic willingly rather than fighting it, it will not mount. The agoraphobic should understand that the cure for agoraphobia does not mean the elimination of anxiety, but instead involves learning techniques to successfully live with anxiety. As she learns not to fear her fears, they will decrease. Daily practice in dealing with fears is the most effective way of overcoming them.

In contrast to desensitization which is done gradually, some therapists use "flooding" which consists of persuading the patient to remain in the stress-producing environment until the anxiety dies down, sometimes several hours. Most patients will overcome the worst of their problem with about eight exposure sessions, a total of twelve hours of exposure.

Reinforcement therapy is also useful in agoraphobia. This therapy is based on the fact that any response which is followed by reinforcement (approval) frequently enough will increase in frequency. The patient who has difficulty shopping may begin by writing a shopping list. With repeated approval from her therapist the problem becomes less. The next phase may consist of having the patient put on her coat and walk to the door. The next step may be opening the door and walking to the car, and so on, until the patient can actually go inside the store and purchase the necessary items.

For any treatment to be effective the agoraphobic must be willing to accept the responsibility for cooperating with treatment and to make a firm commitment to stay with the program. The patient must understand that failure in the program is only a temporary situation, and only she can let it become a permanent behavior pattern. Fears control our lives as much as we are willing to let them; and each of us decides what makes us fearful. We are the cause of our own discomfort.

## TREATMENT

1. Remove all sugar and sugar-containing foods from the diet.
2. Use no "white foods," white rice, white starch, spaghetti, macaroni, other pastas, bread, etc. Use all these foods in their whole grain forms.
3. Use no coffee, tea, colas, chocolate or other caffeine-containing bevzerages or foods.
4. Maintain good posture at all times – sitting, standing, and lying. Once an hour consciously breathe deeply five to ten times. Once daily, take an exercise in breathing as follows: Lift the hands over the head as if grasping a bar located overhead. Breathe as deeply as comfortable. Hold it for a few seconds. Then exhale while bending over at the waist. Let the hands fall down in front crossing the arms in scissors fashion to encourage full expiration. Repeat five times.

5. Wear no tight clothing around the chest or waist.
6. If breathing becomes rapid, consciously slow down and breathe deeply.
7. If a thought producing anxiety occurs, say "stop" audibly. Then switch thoughts to a previously selected topic.
8. Organize a desensitization routine. A sample routine might include practicing the following; Write a grocery list. Walk from the house to the car. This step may need to be repeated several times. Drive from the house to the market. Again repeat if necessary. Walk from the parking lot to the front of the market. If uncomfortable, return to the car and walk to it again several times until you can enter the building. Continue each step in this way until the groceries have been successfully stored in the pantry.
9. Do not allow a failure to discourage you. Begin again with determination, firmness and persistence.
10. Pray for victory. Though you may not know a personal God, millions have obtained help through prayer. It is an effective means of therapy, and by the laws of our spiritual nature, God is enabled to do for us what He cannot do if we do not pray. The benefits of prayer have been demonstrated by such organizations as Alcoholics Anonymous and other self-help groups.

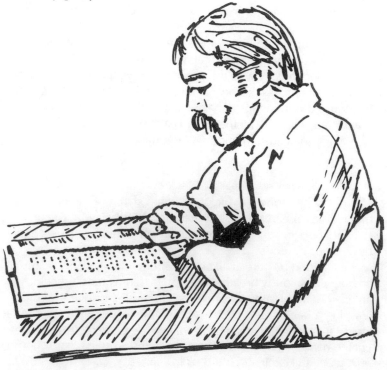

## ANEMIA (IRON DEFICIENCY)

Anemia is not a disease in itself, but rather a laboratory diagnosis indicating a low red blood cell count and below normal hematocrit or hemoglobin levels. (1) There is an insufficient amount of hemoglobin to carry oxygen to the tissues. Iron deficiency anemia, the most common type, occurs when the total body iron level is decreased below normal levels. The body's need for iron may exceed the supply in chronic blood loss, impaired gastrointestinal uptake of iron, pregnancy, menstruation, periods of rapid growth and insufficient uptake.

Most of the cells in the blood are red blood cells. The percentage of red blood cells in the blood is called the hematocrit. The chief function of red blood cells is to carry oxygen from the lungs to the tissues. Oxygen diffuses through the pulmonary membrane into the blood where it enters the cell membrane and combines with the hemoglobin inside the red blood cell. When the red blood cell reaches a tissue capillary the hemoglobin releases the oxygen which diffuses out of the capillary and into the tissues. (32)

*Hematocrit tube,
used to measure
hemoglobin levels*

In the adult, red blood cells are formed in the marrow of bones such as the skull, vertebra, ribs, pelvis, and sternum. In the fetus, red blood cells are formed in the yolk sac, the liver, spleen and the bone marrow, but by birth only the bone marrow continues this task. The rate of red blood cell formation decreases with age, accounting for the frequency of anemia in elderly people.

Several substances including iron, copper, cobalt, nickel, folic acid, and vitamins B-6 and B-12 are necessary for hemoglobin formation.

Red blood cells, also called erythrocytes, are biconcave discs which must twist and fold as they squeeze through the smallest blood vessels. Because of this wear and tear their average lifespan is only about 120 days. With each tick of the clock three million red blood cells in your body die. (34) During their brief lifetime red blood cells make more than 300,000

trips around your body, more than 700 miles, carrying more than 3 quad-
rillion molecules of oxygen to body tissues! (33)

Hemoglobin contains 60 to 70 percent of the iron found in the
human body: 30 to 35 percent is found in iron stores in the liver, spleen,
and bone marrow. Small amounts of iron are found in muscle myoglobin,
blood serum and every cell of the body. (20)

Symptoms of anemia may include easy tiring, headache, dizziness,
ringing in the ears, rapid heart rate, shortness of breath on exertion, abnormal sensations such as burning, prickling, etc.; paleness of the skin and
mucous membranes; sore or smooth tongue, cold sensitivity, poor appetite, lesions at the corners of the mouth and cravings for unusual substances such as starch, clay, or ice. All of these symptoms are due to the blood's
inability to carry adequate oxygen to the body tissues. (2)

Only about five to ten percent of ingested iron is absorbed by the
body, but absorption increases as need increases. Patients with iron deficiency anemia may absorb 45 to 64 percent of iron ingested. (21) The normal adult male has iron stores of approximately 900 mg; the adult female,
who loses iron during pregnancies and menstruation, and generally eats a
diet lower in iron, has stores of only about 300 mg. An average of 20 mg.
of iron is lost in each menstrual cycle, but women who bleed heavily may
lose considerably more.

## TREATMENT

It is absolutely essential that anemia be accurately diagnosed before
embarking on any treatment plan. There are many causes of anemia, some
of which are quite serious or life-threatening. This is especially true in post-
menopausal women who do not have an obvious reason for blood loss.

The indiscriminate taking of supplements and vitamins may mask potentially serious conditions. It is assumed in this section that the reader has
had an accurate diagnosis of anemia, since otherwise he could not even
know of it. If he only suspects anemia, we would urge a complete history,
physical examination, and appropriate diagnostic studies by a qualified
physician.

1. Diet is the mainstay of anemia treatment. It should be high in unre-
   fined and unprocessed foods, in as near their natural state as possible.
   The following suggestions may be helpful:
   A. Avoid milk and other diary products as these decrease iron ab-
      sorption from other foods. (6)
   B. Avoid hot or spicy foods if sore tongue or mouth is present.
   C. Tea and coffee decrease iron absorption and should be avoided.
      (3) Orange juice increases the absorption.
   D. Apricots, peaches and prunes, dried or fresh, contain factors very
      favorable for hemoglobin development. Raisins, fresh grapes, and
      dried or fresh apples are slightly less effective. (4)

E. Whole wheat flour and oatmeal are effective in hemoglobin regeneration. (5)
F. Use a diet high in fresh and raw fruits and vegetables which are high in vitamin C. Vitamin C is necessary for the absorption of iron from the digestive tract.
G. Spinach, lettuce and tomato mixture, asparagus, lettuce, and broccoli all encourage hemoglobin regeneration. The lettuce and tomato mixture was slightly more effective than the lettuce alone. (7)
H. Green leafy vegetables are high in iron and should be used frequently. Foods low in iron have a noticeable lack of color.
I. Yeast and wheat germ are reported to be high in iron. Other vegetarian foods high in iron include whole grains, beets and beet greens, cabbage, celery, parsley, dates, cherries, figs, and pears.
J. Phosphates and antacids decrease iron absorption. (23) Phytates, present in whole grains, are said to decrease iron absorption, but studies done on women eating a diet very high in chapatis from whole grains show no lack of iron.
K. Iron absorption from soybeans has been shown to be greater than that from spinach. (24)
L. Eggs decrease the uptake of iron from some foods. (25)
M. Iron is present in bananas in sufficient amounts to induce some hemoglobin regeneration. (34)

2. Rest lowers the oxygen requirements and reduces stress on the heart and lungs. Anemic people should be encouraged to rest or nap during the day and to get adequate nighttime sleep. Resting without a pillow increases circulation of blood and oxygen to the brain and may help relieve dizziness. (2)

3. Special mouth care may be necessary because anemic patients often have a sore mouth or tongue. Teeth should be cleaned with a soft-bristle toothbrush. Rinsing the mouth every two hours and lubricating the lips with mineral oil or petrolatum may prevent cracking or dryness. (2)

4. Patients with anemia have poor blood circulation and must be protected from both chilling and burns. Warm clothing and adequate blankets at night increase patient comfort.

5. Ferrous sulfate and other iron compounds are often given in anemia, but they have been shown to have toxic effects. They destroy vitamin E (26), increase oxygen need, damage unsaturated fatty acids, and destroy carotene and vitamins A and C. (8-11) Iron compounds may induce liver damage, particularly when the patient has a poor appetite. (12) Iron salts taken during pregnancy may further increase the fetus' need for oxygen, induce miscarriage, premature or post-mature births

(13-14), and may produce malformation or mental deficiency in infants. (15, 16)

Iron is so readily available in unrefined foods that a normal person eating an unrefined diet should not develop iron deficiency anemia. The iron in unrefined foods is never toxic. "No effective iron preparation is free from causing gastric or intestinal irritation." (28)

6. A number of drugs destroy vitamin E (17) and others inactivate nutrients needed to produce blood cells (18) inducing anemia. Several insecticides are known to damage bone marrow (19) preventing the development of new blood cells. Food additives and artificial sweeteners are also suspect and should be avoided. Tetracycline binds iron and diminishes absorption. (27)

7. Exercise stimulates the bone marrow to produce blood cells and promotes absorption of iron from the intestine. Vigorous exercise increases the rate of red cell production. (32) A well-trained athlete may have a red blood cell count of 6.5 million per cubic mm., while inactive persons, whose tissues receive little oxygen, may have a red blood cell count as low as 3 million. (32) A simple lack of exercise is probably the most common cause of mild anemia, and a person with anemia from this source will continue to have anemia even if treated with all the substances known to be necessary for red blood cell formation, including iron! (32)

8. A short cold bath may stimulate the bone marrow. Water temperature may be 40 to 90 degrees; the greater the cold the less time spent in the bath, e. g. one-half minute at 40 to 50 degrees, one minute at 60 to 70 degrees; two minutes at 70-80 degrees, three minutes at 80 to 85 degrees; and three and one half minutes at 90 degrees. Frictioning the skin with a brush or coarse washcloth makes the bath more tolerable, as does cold splashing water on the face before jumping quickly into the tub or shower.

9. Vitamin D assists in blood making. Daily sun exposure will supply adequate amounts, even if the exposure is for only ten minutes and the sunshine strikes directly only a small patch of skin no larger than the face.

10. Cooking food in iron pots contributes significantly to the iron content of foods. (22)

11. Water from deep wells or bore holes may contain higher amounts of iron than city water.

12. A cold mitten friction may be very effective in stimulating blood cell production. To do a cold mitten friction wring a friction mitt or heavy washcloth out of water 40 to 70 degrees F. Rub the entire body, one section at a time, briskly for five to eight seconds. Dry quickly and proceed to the next area. Expose only the part being treated to avoid chilling. (30) (See HOME REMEDIES for more information on cold mitten friction.)

13. Massage may be very useful in anemia. In one case there were 4,500,000 red cells per cu. mm. before massage and 6,400,000 afterwards. (29)

## ATHEROSCLEROSIS AND ARTERIOSCLEROSIS

The word atherosclerosis comes from two Greek words "athere" which means "mush" or "porridge" and "skleros" meaning "hard." The atherosclerotic lesion begins as a soft deposit in the arterial blood vessel and hardens as it ages. These deposits or lesions are called plaques. They grow gradually, thickening the walls of the artery, and narrowing the opening through which the blood can flow. The plaque is made up of a combination of substances including cholesterol, lipoproteins, fatty acids, calcium deposits, fibrous scar tissue, and blood. These plaques cause a loss of the elasticity of the blood vessel wall. (83)

If a blood clot forms in these narrowed blood vessels and cuts off the blood supply to the heart a heart attack occurs. A stroke is the result of occlusion of the blood flow to the brain.

Most patients with coronary artery disease have elevated blood cholesterol levels. The typical American may receive 800 to 1000 mg. of cholesterol each day from meat, eggs, whole milk and milk products. A single egg contains approximately 250 mg. of cholesterol! As the dietary intake of cholesterol increases, the blood cholesterol levels generally increase.

Saturated fats were discovered to increase serum cholesterol, but fats made up primarily of polyunsaturated fatty acids may decrease serum cholesterol. (82) Saturated fats are primarily of animal origin although coconut oil is an exception. Polyunsaturated fats are primarily of vegetable origin. (83)

Atherosclerosis is considered a degenerative disease, but recently fatty streaks in the major arteries of the body have been observed in the first years of life. (83) Some researchers feel this is due to feeding infants cow's milk rather than breast milk.

Atherosclerosis is the commonest form of arterial disease in the United States today. It is a generalized arterial disease which rarely occurs in the absence of arteriosclerosis. Arteriosclerosis is sometimes called "hardening of the arteries." Atherosclerosis most commonly affects the main arteries, generally in a patchy manner. When it is in the limbs it is usually present elsewhere in the body. Atherosclerosis occurs more frequently in the lower than the upper limbs. The lesions cause narrowing of the blood vessels, resulting in reduced blood flow.

Atherosclerosis is apparently a disease of multiple causes; a number of risk factors have been identified including elevated cholesterol and triglyceride levels, high fat diet, smoking, obesity, emotional stress, lack of exercise, and diseases such as diabetes and hypertension. (69) Estrogen and other hormones have a potent effect on atherogenesis, estrogens slowing down the rate of development. Genetic factors also appear to be important.

Atherosclerosis is the most frequent cause of death in persons over age 65. Over 50 percent of all people between 60 and 70 will die due to some manifestation of atherosclerosis. Myocardial infarction (heart attack) or cerebral vascular accident (stroke) is frequently a clinical manifestation of atherosclerosis. Intermittent claudication (pain in the legs on walking) is commonly reported.

## TREATMENT

1. Refined sugar has been shown to produce increased serum cholesterol levels leading to atherosclerotic heart disease. Both sucrose and fructose are atherogenic. (60)
2. Dietary animal proteins demonstrate a strong positive correlation with mortality from cardiovascular disease in human studies. (61) Rabbits given casein absorb cholesterol from the intestine more readily than rabbits fed soy protein.
3. Fibers of fruits, legumes and vegetables decrease blood fats and increase excretion of bile acids. Wheat bran and other particulate fibers do not seem as effective in this role as are those found in fruits, vegetables, and legumes. (62)
4. Rabbits given garlic oil with cholesterol-containing foods showed decreased atheromatous changes in the aorta. (64) Onion apparently acts in a similar manner. (66)
5. Peanut oil and coconut oil have been shown to be atherogenic (in feeding experiments containing massive quantities of sugar – 25%) despite the fact that they are vegetable oils. (65, 67) Vegetable oils are generally considered to be non-atherogenic contrasted to animal fats which are atherogenic.
6. Refined sugar and white flour fed to mice produced atherosclerosis. (68) Use a low sugar diet, and whole grain flours.
7. Olive oil has a beneficial effect on cholesterol. (70) A group of ten patients with artery disease showed an average drop of 26 percent in blood lipids after four months on olive oil, and the cholesterol levels dropped over 14 percent. A diet containing no free fats would be the diet of choice for most people with artery disease. See SUE'S KITCHEN for suggestions.
8. Eggplant has been shown to be effective in lowering cholesterol levels. It apparently breaks down into compounds that bind with cholesterol and carry it out of the digestive tract. (71)

9. Eight men with high cholesterol levels were given about one-half cup dry measure of beans per day. Three weeks later their cholesterol levels had dropped by an average of 20 percent. Interestingly, the atherogenic LDH (low density lipoproteins) were decreased, while the desirable high density lipoprotein (HDL) fraction remained unchanged. (72)

10. A strict vegetarian diet is helpful. Strict vegetarians have lower levels of cholesterol than do meat eaters or lacto-ovo-vegetarians who use milk. and eggs. (73)

11. Many people have switched to skim milk to lower their cholesterol levels, but studies at the University of Wisconsin at Madison revealed that skim milk actually increased blood levels of cholesterol. (74)

12. Chromium was found to lower cholesterol levels in rabbits given a high cholesterol diet, and they showed a 50 percent reduction of coronary artery plaques. (75) Brewer's yeast and whole grains are good sources of chromium.

13. The typical American heavy supper may contribute to arteriosclerosis, according to Dr. Paul B. Roen, senior director of the Hollywood Presbyterian Medical Center Clinic for the Study of Arteriosclerosis. Dr. Roen observes that the large amounts of animal fats in the supper are digested primarily during the sleeping hours while the overall basal metabolic rate is low and blood circulation is sluggish. This causes cholesterol to be deposited in arteries that may be already narrowed by plaque. (79) A light, low-fat supper, eaten several hours before bedtime would reduce the level of fat in the blood during sleeping hours. The ideal supper is a small meal of plain fruit and plain bread or other whole grain.

14. Premature arteriosclerosis may be induced by irradiation. (80) X-ray exposure should be kept to a minimum.

15. A regular exercise program such as walking will generally help the patient feel better. This may be due to increased collateral circulation in the limbs.

16. Overweight patients should begin a weight reduction program to bring the weight back to ideal or slightly below ideal. Obesity 20 percent or more above ideal weight carries a significantly increased risk of atherosclerotic disease. A general rule of thumb for average American weight is that one calculates 100 pounds for the first five feet, and five pounds for each inch of one's height thereafter for a woman, and seven pounds for each inch thereafter if a man.

17. Cigarette smoking decreases cutaneous blood flow and may influence blood vessel disability. It also increases blood circulating lipids and alters metabolism of these substances. (69) A group of smokers who stopped smoking experienced a rapid and significant increase in HDL levels (the beneficial blood fats). (76) Smokers who are also diabetics

are more than twice as likely to develop arteriosclerosis as are non-smoking diabetics. (78)

18. The feet should be given special attention as the decreased blood flow may retard healing. Shoes and slippers should fit properly. The feet should be washed using warm water, and dried gently and thoroughly. Clean wool or cotton socks should be worn daily. Avoid going barefoot as this increases risk of injury to the feet.

19. Eliminate all items of clothing such as garters, girdles, hosiery, etc. which are constricting and may cause reduced blood flow.

20. Use an electric blanket rather than hot water bottles or heating pads as these are more likely to cause burns. People with decreased blood flow are more susceptible to burns and less sensitive to extreme temperatures.

21. Dress to keep all extremities warm. Cold limbs discourage blood circulation. Cholesterol was significantly increased in a group of rats fed a stock diet but kept in a cold environment. (63) This phenomenon is probably due to stress, at least in part.

22. Hypertension (high blood pressure) produces physical stress in the walls of the arteries and results in aggravation and acceleration of atherosclerosis. Hypertension apparently increases the susceptibility of both large and small arteries to atherosclerosis. (64) Hypertension should be carefully treated if present.

23. Glucose intolerance may cause a 100 percent excess risk of atherosclerosis. (77) Blood sugar levels should be carefully controlled.

## CATARACTS

A cataract is a cloudy or opaque area in the lens of the eye. The lens, a small, oval tissue located behind the pupil and iris, helps focus light onto the retina. Usually the lens is clear but if it becomes clouded with a cataract the passage of light is obstructed and vision may be impaired.

Cataracts vary from very small to large cloudy areas that cause marked loss of vision. They can develop over a period of years or within a few months.

In the United States alone cataracts are diagnosed in approximately five million people a year. (35) Symptoms are gradually failing vision, hazy, fuzzy, or blurred vision, change in the color of the pupil, seeing better without glasses, the need for frequent change in eyeglass prescriptions, a feeling of having film over the eyes, and seeing rings or halos around lights. (36) Cataracts can be congenital, or caused by injury, disease, or aging.

Congenital cataract is more likely if the mother has had rubella during the first three months of pregnancy or if the infant has galactosemia (an inherited disorder of galactose metabolism). Congenital cataracts are generally stationary and do not progress. They are usually associated with other congenital abnormalities.

Traumatic cataracts are caused by blunt or penetrating injury that ruptures the anterior lens capsule. This causes the lens to absorb aqueous humor. The lens becomes cloudy and must be removed to restore sight. Exposure to harmful chemicals may also induce traumatic cataracts.

Diseases known to cause cataracts are diabetes, hypoparathyroidism, galactosemia, Down's, Lowe's and Werner's syndromes, (37) and atopic dermatitis. Cataracts may occur as a complication of uveitis, iritis, glaucoma, tumors, chorioretinitis, detached retina, severe myopia, or retinitis pigmentosa.

Infrared rays from intense heat, ionizing radiation, and chemical agents can also produce cataracts. Jewelers who sit for hours daily for many years, with the eyes becoming heated from the light placed only an inch or two from the eyes, are prone to develop cataracts from the prolonged heating of the eyes.

Senile cataracts are probably the most common type. The three kinds of senile cataract are nuclear, cortical, and posterior subcapsular. The lens may take on a brownish tinge with a nuclear cataract, and as it progresses may appear even black. The nucleus hardens and patients may suddenly discover that they can read even without their glasses. However, vision worsens as the cataract progresses and patients become unable to see even with glasses. This type of cataract usually grows slowly. Cortical cataracts involve the outer layer of the lens within the capsule, while posterior subcapsular cataracts appear on the back surface of the lens. (36)

Chemically, cataract formation is characterized by a reduction in oxygen uptake, and an initial increase in water content which is followed by dehydration. (37)

## PREVENTION

1. Diabetes has been associated with cataract formation. (38) The longer the duration of the disease, the greater the risk of cataract.
2. Galactose-fed rats develop elevated blood sugar levels, inducing cataract formation. Galactose is apparently four times as effective as glucose in producing cataracts. (39, 40) Galactose comes from milk sugar.
3. Oral hypoglycemic agents have been significantly associated with cataract formation. (38) Diabinese, Dymelor, Orinase, (Tolbutamide), and Tolinase are oral antidiabetic medications.
4. Anorexia nervosa has been associated with cataract formation. (41)
5. High blood levels of glucose or xylose produce cataracts. (40) Use a low sugar diet, and avoid the use of sugar substitutes.
6. Corticosteroid therapy has been shown to induce cataracts. (42) The risk increases as the dosage and length of administration increase.
7. Some studies have suggested a relationship between sunlight and cataract formation. An Australian study found a higher incidence of cataracts in Aborigines living in areas of high UV irradiation than counter-

parts living in areas of low UV irradiation. Not only are those living in areas of high UV irradiation more likely to develop cataracts; but to develop them earlier in life, and more likely to be blind or visually handicapped by them. (43) The authors suggest that the use of sunglasses may be helpful in preventing cataracts. Other sources of radiation including x-rays and microwaves may induce cataracts, as may intense heat.

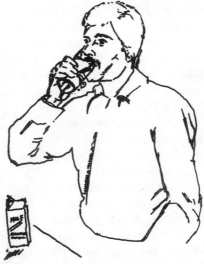

*Galactose in milk can induce cataract formation*

8. A high level of phospholipids (fats) in the blood is associated with increased cataract risk. (46)
9. A number of drugs have been associated with cataracts: Barbiturates, antihypertensive drugs, monoamine oxidase inhibitors, tricyclic antidepressants, phenothiazines, (55) corticosteroids (56) allopurinol (57) tetracycline and other broad spectrum antibiotics, sulphonamides, antihistamines, (58) pilocarpine, anticholinesterase agents (44) myleran and other radiomimetic drugs, oral contraceptives, pontocaine, ergot, the morphine group, streptozotocine, paradichlorobenzol (used in deodorants, moth repellents, and insecticides) and many other drugs. (47)
10. Senile cataracts are associated with high blood pressure. (46) There is also an association between antihypertensive drugs and cataracts.
11. Naphthalene (mothballs) has been shown to induce cataracts. (47)
12. Dr. Barton L. Hodes of Chicago feels that cigarette smoking is, if not directly cataractogenic, at least a factor contributing to the premature development of lens opacities. (49)
13. Hair dye has been shown to cause cataracts. Eighty-nine percent of a

group of hair dye users had lens changes while only twenty-three percent of non-users showed changes. (50)

14. Lactose (milk sugar) has been demonstrated to induce cataracts. All of a group of laboratory animals given a 70 percent lactose ration showed lens changes and 68 percent showed mature bilateral cataracts. (51) There is a greater likelihood of cataracts in old age in those persons who tolerate milk well in youth (generally white Americans and others of Northern European extraction). The mechanism is that those who tolerate milk well are capable of splitting milk sugar so that galactose is absorbed from the intestinal tract. Those who use milk regularly get "repeated small galactose challenges, accumulation of galactitol in the lens, and a greater likelihood of developing cataracts." (287)

15. Lying down after meals encourages fat build-up in the blood, decreasing blood flow in the small blood vessels, encouraging a condition which may increase the risk of cataracts.

16. Deep breathing exercises stimulate circulation. Therefore some moderate exercise after meals would be helpful in reducing cataract formation. Exercise has been shown to delay cataract formation. (52)

17. Cataracts occur with greater frequency and at an earlier age in allergic than in non-allergic people. (53)

18. Stressed laboratory guinea pigs developed cataracts, while non-stressed guinea pigs living under otherwise similar conditions did not. (54) Stress can result from chilling of the body, biochemical imbalances, disease, as well as from emotional factors.

19. Methylmercury in fish may cause clouding of the lens, contributing to cataract development. Optometrist Ben Lane noted that his cataract patients liked seafood, while those who didn't like fish were clear-eyed. A study of 17 patients revealed that the cataract patients had eaten salt water fish or shellfish at least once a week on the average, but those cataract-free reported using these foods an average of once every five weeks. The cataract patients showed far higher concentrations of mercury in their hair. Dr. Lane's study showed that the presence of 2.3 ppm or more of mercury in hair samples was related to a 23-fold increase in the risk of cataracts. Dr. Lane encourages his patients to eat such foods as garlic and pectin-rich food such as apples to help remove the mercury, and to receive adequate, while avoiding excessive amounts of vitamins A, C, and E. (288)

## CERVICITIS

Cervicitis in an inflammation of the cervix. There are two forms of cervicitis – acute and chronic. Chronic cervicitis is the most common pathologic condition of the cervix. (117) Acute cervicitis often progresses to the chronic stage and symptoms may be so minimal that the disease may be undetected and untreated for a long period of time. Leukorrhea (a whitish, sticky discharge from the vagina and uterine cavity) may be the only symptom. Pain is generally not present unless the infection spreads upward to involve the uterus or nearby pelvic organs.

Pathogens introduced by intercourse or by douching may induce cervicitis. Cervicitis may occur after childbirth or may be caused by an infection of a cervical tear. An alkaline vaginal pH makes infection more likely. (118) The tissues are constantly irritated in chronic cervicitis, and some studies suggest that the irritation may lead to cancer.

## TREATMENT

1. Hot foot baths taken every four hours are very beneficial. The blood flow to vaginal and cervical tissues is increased reflexively by the hot foot bath.

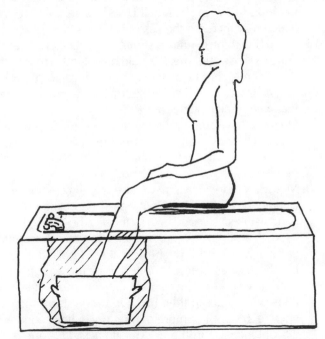

*Hot foot baths every four hours can be beneficial in cervicitis*

2. Douching with an appropriate solution can be curative.
   A.  For yeast infections (found more in women with a family history of diabetes), use hot soda water douches once daily for ten to thirty days. Use one teaspoon of baking soda to a quart of water.
   B.  For trichomonas infection, use hot vinegar douches. Put one to four tablespoons of ordinary vinegar in one quart of hot water. Douche once daily for ten to thirty days.

C. For ordinary bacterial infections use a hot garlic water douche. Whirl one clove of garlic in one cup of boiling water in a blender. Add three more cups of boiling water to the blender and allow to "cook" while cooling. Use once daily for ten to thirty days.

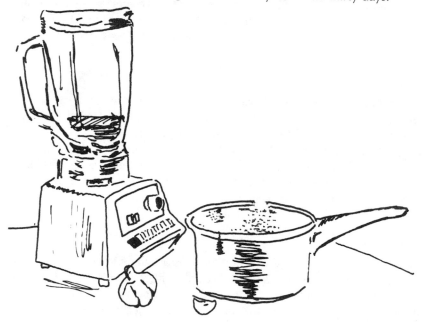

*Blend clove of garlic with 4 cups hot water for garlic douche*

3. Hot baths are very good for cervicitis. Take a hot bath for 20 minutes while keeping the head cool, once daily for seven to ten days. Follow each bath with a brief cool shower and a 20-30 minute rest in bed.
4. Since many cases of cervicitis are caused by cold extremities, wear enough warm underwear and stockings to keep the feet as warm as the forehead.

## CHICKENPOX (VARICELLA ZOSTER)

Chickenpox is an acute disease common in childhood. The disease is spread by direct contact with infected lesions (pox) and by airborne droplets. It is communicable from one to two days before the rash develops until all the blister-like lesions have crusted, an average of five or six days.

It occurs most commonly between the ages of two and eight in the temperate zones of the world, with its peak incidence on beginning school. It is one of the most contagious of all the infectious diseases. Most cases occur in the winter and spring.

Onset is generally 14 to 21 days after exposure. Young children exhibit low grade fever, rash, and a general feeling of discomfort, but older people may have a prodrome of fever, muscle aches and headache for one to two days prior to the onset of the lesions. Lesions appear initially on the trunk and scalp and progress rapidly over 12 to 24 hours to crusted lesions.

Lesions occur in crops and the patient may experience two to four crops in two to six days. There may be lesions in all stages in the same area of the body. The fever is related to the severity of the rash.

The blister-like lesions may also occur in the mouth, vagina, conjunctiva and pharynx.

Chickenpox is generally worse in adults than in children, with more severe rash, higher fever and a higher rate of complications. Deformities in the baby have been observed in some cases in which the pregnant mother was infected with the virus during the first four months of pregnancy.

Herpes zoster (shingles) is a reactivation of a latent chickenpox infection. Susceptible persons may acquire chickenpox from patients with shingles, and at least one documented case is recorded of a person getting shingles from a case of chickenpox.

## TREATMENT

1. Itching may be relieved with applications of calamine lotion, moist baking soda, honey or starch baths. Nails should be kept short and clean to minimize the possibility of infection from scratching. Scratching in young children may be discouraged by having them wear mittens or gloves, especially at night. Apply pressure to the area instead of scratching.
2. There is no evidence that antibiotics or corticosteroids are useful in chickenpox (84) and they should not be used.
3. Aspirin should not be used to lower the fever as about ten percent of cases of Reyes syndrome occur following chickenpox. (84) Reyes syndrome is a catastrophic disease in children, often causing death or an irreversible coma. The course is as follows: the fever of chickenpox develops for which aspirin is given, some improvement occurs for a day or two, followed by a sharp change for the worse, rapidly developing coma, and a high likelihood of death.
4. Skin care includes a daily tepid bath and a daily change of clothes and linens. It is important to protect against chilling while bathing and at all other times, as chickenpox pneumonia can develop following exposure, even in the convalescent stage. Oatmeal baths may be soothing. For an oatmeal bath put one pound of uncooked oatmeal, or one heaping cup of uncooked rolled oats ground fine in a blender, in a bag made of two thicknesses of some material similar to old sheeting or gauze. Float the bag in the bath water or hang it from the faucet and let the water entering the tub run through it. Use hot water first to soften the

oatmeal. The bag may be used to gently sponge the body. Pat dry rather than rubbing dry after the bath.

5. Saline rinses and gargles may be soothing to mouth lesions and saline soaks (1 level teaspoon salt to 1 pint (two cups) of water) may be used for perineal lesions.
6. Children should be kept out of school until all lesions have crusted.
7. At the onset of the disease a deep, warm, 15 minute bath will encourage the pox to come out rapidly. Keep the heat cool.
8. Use a light, fat-free, sugar-free diet.
9. Avoid constipation at all times.

## CONJUNCTIVITIS

Conjunctivitis is an inflammation of the conjunctiva, the mucous membrane which lines the inner surface of the eyelid and continues over the surface of the eyeball. The inflammation may be due to bacterial or viral infection, or physical or chemical injury.

Acute bacterial conjunctivitis is sometimes called "pink eye, or "sore eyes." This condition is highly contagious and often occurs in groups of schoolchildren. Conjunctivitis is probably the most common eye disease in the Western Hemisphere.

Symptoms include redness, swelling, tearing and discomfort. There may be a discharge from the eye. Generally a thin, watery discharge suggests that the conjunctivitis is of viral origin, a white, stringy discharge suggests allergic origin and a discharge containing pus suggests conjunctivitis of a bacterial origin. (85)

The conjunctiva has relatively few pain fibers, therefore a sensation of discomfort, burning, or scratchiness is characteristic. Itching and light sensitivity may also be present, especially in allergic conjunctivitis.

## TREATMENT

1. Charcoal poultices should be applied overnight. Mix powdered charcoal with water sufficient to make a thick paste, and spread it over a piece of flannel or muslin larger than the inflamed area of the eye. Place this over the eye. Cover with a piece of plastic or similar material and hold in place with an ace bandage wrapped lightly around the head. The bandage should not be so tight that it puts pressure on the eyeballs, but it must be snug enough to hold the compress in place overnight. Remove it in the morning, disposing of the compress in a manner to avoid spreading the infection.
2. Charcoal slurry water eye drops may be used during the day. To make the drops boil one cup of water with one-fourth teaspoon salt and one teaspoon powdered charcoal. When cool, strain through several layers of cheesecloth. Using a dropper, put four or five drops of the clear fluid in the affected eye every two hours.

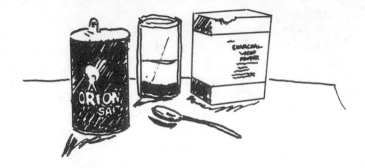

3. During acute conjunctivitis ice cold compresses may be applied. Wring a washcloth from ice water, and apply to the eye. Renew every two to three minutes for half an hour, discontinue for 30 to 60 minutes, then repeat for another half an hour.
4. Hot and cold applications may be applied every four hours in cases of chronic conjunctivitis. Wring a washcloth out of very hot (but not boiling) water and apply to the eye for two minutes, alternating with another cloth wrung from ice water and applied for 30 seconds, with alternations for 15 minutes.
5. Use a sugar-free, low-fat diet to assist the body in overcoming the infection.
6. Do not place a patch on the eye as it may promote bacterial growth, (86) but for light sensitivity dark glasses may be worn for a day or two. The patient may be more comfortable in a darkened room because of light sensitivity.
7. Wash the hands carefully after each treatment. Do not touch the other eye to avoid spreading the infection. If the eyes itch, the eyelids should be tightly closed, as tightly as the child can squeeze the eyelids, and then the eyes can be moved from side to side by looking from right to left with the eyelids closed. This is a gentle massage. Bathtowels and washcloths should be laundered frequently and sun dried. They should not be shared by others.
8. Corticosteroids reduce the resistance of the eye to bacteria and should not be used, (86) either in drops or by mouth.
9. The eye is ten times more sensitive to allergens than the skin and allergic conjunctivitis is common. It may be associated with tree pollen, grasses, weeds, molds, house dust, animal dander, and chemicals and drugs, including cosmetics. These substances should be avoided by people with known sensitivities. (87) Allergic conjunctivitis is commonly seasonal and may be manifested by intense itching, tearing and swelling. Cold compresses may be soothing. (88)

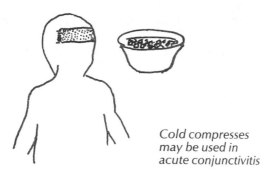

*Cold compresses
may be used in
acute conjunctivitis*

10. Vernal conjunctivitis may recur for many years. It generally begins in the prepubertal years and may begin in the spring and last through to autumn. Allergy seems to play a role in its development. (88) Fever therapy has been shown effective in treating it. (89) Two or three treatments may be sufficient. Sit in a tub of hot water at 103 to 110 degrees F. for a period of time sufficient to bring the oral temperature up to about 101 degrees. Babies under age three need three minutes, and children over three need one minute for each year of their age. After the temperature is above 100 keep the head cool by keeping a cold washcloth on the throat or forehead.

11. Saline irrigations may be used to rinse discharges from the eyes. Add two level teaspoons of salt to a quart of water to make physiologic saline.

## CONSTIPATION

Constipation is one of the most common problems of modern times. It is a disorder of the colon producing infrequent or difficult emptying of the bowels. The stools are hard and dry. Other symptoms may be dull headache, abdominal discomfort, lack of energy, poor appetite, and low back pain. The word "constipation" comes from a Latin word meaning "crowded together." It indicates an incomplete or too infrequent emptying of the bowels.

When eating a balanced diet, three meals daily, the amount of feces excreted each day varies from three to seven ounces. The more fiber in the diet the larger the amount of feces and softer the consistency. Concentrated foods such as meats, sugar and cheese lead to smaller quantities of feces of harder consistency. Africans on their fiber-rich diet may pass five to ten times the amount of feces passed by the "normal" American.

Most authorities agree that bowel movements which come at the same time every day are more effective than irregular movements. The most beneficial time for a bowel movement is probably the early morning before or soon after breakfast.

The person with the best bowel health probably has a bowel movement after each meal, but some people have bowel movements only once or twice a week.

Factors commonly associated with constipation are too little fiber in foods, too little liquid, too little physical exercise, and emotional tension.

## PREVENTION AND TREATMENT

1. A diet high in fiber-containing foods is essential in constipation. Whole grain cereals, leafy vegetables, roots and fresh or cooked fruit are all good sources of fiber. Fiber is not digested and stimulates the colon by its bulk.

   Bran is often used to increase fiber intake. One to four heaping tablespoons of bran flakes are often adequate to normalize bowel habits. Coarse bran has a greater water-holding capacity and is probably preferable in the treatment of bowel problems. (111) Raw bran produces faster intestinal transit than does cooked bran. (115) Corn bran has been shown to be significantly better than wheat bran in relieving constipation. (112)

2. Most of the ill effects of constipation are caused by its treatment. (116) Laxatives pass from your mouth through over 20 feet of the digestive system before leaving the body. These sensitive tissues are irritated by the laxative on its way to the site of action. Adverse effects of laxatives include potassium loss, weakening of intestinal motility and severe kidney damage. It has been known since A.D. 100 that purgatives can cause constipation by irritating the bowels and paralyzing them. (105)

   A 1957 article in *Science News* suggests that the common use of purgatives leads to appendicitis. (106)

   Mineral oil is probably the most harmful of all laxatives. It decreases calcium and phosphorus absorption (99) and absorbs vitamins A, D, E, and K, as well as carotene. Continued use of mineral oil may lead to cancer of the colon and bowel.

3. A relationship has been shown between obesity and constipation. (114) If overweight, reduce the body weight at least to average. A woman may allow 100 pounds for the first five feet in height and five pounds for each inch over five feet. Men may add seven pounds for each inch over five feet.

4. A small cold enema is often useful in retraining the bowel to good elimination habits. Inject one bulb syringe (ear irrigation syringe from the drugstore) of cold tap water into the rectum, hold for one minute, and expel. A bowel movement will generally follow. Use this treatment at the same time every day to establish a pattern of regularity.

5. Senna tea may be used on occasion. Add one-half teaspoon of the leaves to one cup of boiling water, allow to steep for 10 to 15 minutes,

strain, and drink. Using senna too frequently can cause the laxative habit.

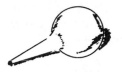

*Bulb syringe*

6. Four to six olives may be eaten with each meal.
7. Abdominal massage has been reported effective in the relief of many cases of constipation. One physician reports that rolling a tennis ball along the line of the colon cured a case of constipation after six weeks. (110) Another method of massage is to apply quick (but not jerky) rocking "punches" with the heel of the hand, alternating the pressure from the right hand applied to the right abdomen with that from the left, in a ball-bouncing effect.

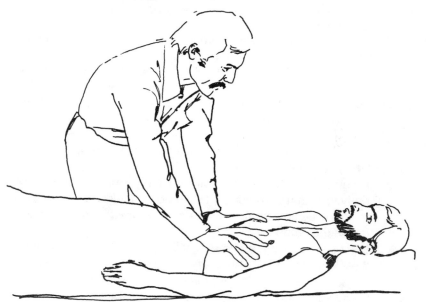

8. A short cold bath may be quite helpful. See the section on Anemia for the procedure.
9. Animal protein should be kept low to discourage intestinal putrefaction. (100) All animal products are low in fiber and tend to be constipating.
10. Geoffry Evans, M.D., in a British publication, *Medical Treatment*, states that fatigue may be a cause of constipation. (101)
11. Hurried and irregular meals may contribute to poor function. (104)

12. All decongestants and antihistamines are drying agents by their nature and may cause the stool to become dryer than normal. Diet pills, pain-killers, amphetamines, and cough preparations containing codeine may adversely affect bowel function. Certain other drugs, prescription and over-the-counter, may cause constipation. (98)

13. Exercise may be helpful in constipation. (102) Walking increases circulation, strengthens the heart and exercises the abdominal muscles, all of which are important to good bowel function.

    Certain exercises are reported helpful if done consistently over a period of time. To do them only a short while, then stop them, will bring on a tightness and perhaps mild physical depression. Begin an exercise program gently, and gradually increase intensity.

    A. Sit on a surface high enough to allow the feet to dangle. Relax completely, allowing the head to fall down on the chest, arms to hang limply at the side, etc. Straighten up with shoulders and head back, chest out, and back arched. Extend the arms to the sides. Hold the position a short time, relax, and repeat the procedure until tired.

    B. Stand on one leg and swing the other leg out and then far back. After five or ten times alternate legs.

    C. Stand with the hands on the hips and rotate the trunk in a circular motion without moving the hips or bending the knees.

    D. Standing, bend over to touch your toes with your fingertips. As you bend tighten the abdominal muscles, hold for a few seconds, and relax.

    E. Lying flat on the back, and moving the legs as one would to ride a bicycle is helpful.

    F. Lie on your back with your hands behind your head. Raise your body to a sitting position and then slowly lower yourself back to the floor. Begin with five sit-ups each morning and gradually increase the number.

    G. Lying on the floor grasp your right knee with both hands and pull it back to rest against your chest. Slowly inhale and exhale while lifting your head to rest your forehead against the knee. Hold the position for a few seconds, and return to the original position. Repeat with the left leg.

    H. Lie on the back, raise the legs as high as possible 10 or 20 times. Repeat morning and evening.

14. Proper toilet position may make bowel evacuation easier. Placing your feet on a small stool is helpful. Ideally the thighs should be against the abdomen, and the higher the stool the closer the thighs come to the abdomen. Leaning forward will bring the abdomen closer to the thighs.

15. Overeating leads to constipation and should be avoided. (115)

16. Milk is a common cause of constipation. (103) A group of young women who eliminated milk and added fruit and vegetable fiber to their diet returned to normal bowel habits of elimination.

   Other foods which encourage constipation due to low fiber content include other dairy products such as cottage cheese, yogurt, and cheese; eggs, fish, poultry, meat, juices, white breads, canned and packaged powdered foods, spices, soda, ice cream, and such items as cookies, cakes, and pies.

17. Some foods are known to have a laxative action. Prunes are probably the most commonly known of these foods, but apples, figs, licorice, raw spinach, and strawberries are all reported to have a laxative action. (107) Prunes contain dihydroxyphenylistan which apparently stimulates intestinal motility. (115) Bananas, apples, and other fruits contain a substance called pectin which takes up a large amount of water. As the pectin moves through the digestive tract it draws bacteria and other debris away from the intestinal wall. It may also possess a healing effect which soothes irritated bowel membranes and restores muscle tone. (115) Figs contain both fiber and pectin and the tiny seeds act as a mild stimulant to the intestines. (115) Soybean sprouts are reported to have laxative properties. (115)

18. Constipation is a common problem during pregnancy, particularly during the latter part. This may be due to pressure on the digestive tract from the growing fetus. (108)

19. Avoid all clothing which constricts the abdomen. Clothing should not leave a red mark on the skin.

20. Adequate fluid intake is essential in the prevention of constipation. (109) Six to eight glasses of water daily are recommended. A glass of hot water before breakfast may stimulate a bowel movement by means of the gastrocolic reflex. Hot or cold fluids are more effective than tepid ones. (101)

21. Tea has been shown to induce constipation. (113)

## CROUP (LARYNGOTRACHEOBRONCHITIS)

Croup is an inflammation or infection of the larynx (vocal cords), trachea (windpipe) and bronchi. It may be caused by a virus, by bacteria, or an allergy. Bacterial croup almost always follows a cold or other apparently mild upper respiratory infection. Parainfluenza viruses are the most common cause of croup (91) but adenoviruses, rhinoviruses and respiratory syncytial virus may also cause croup.

Croup is most common during the winter months. The age range for croup is generally three months to three years, with the peak incidence between nine and eighteen months. Older children may occasionally be affected. Viral croup is more common in boys than in girls.

The typical case of croup presents with a history of a cold for a day or two, a harsh, barking cough, hoarseness, low grade fever, and harsh, high-pitched respiratory sounds.

## TREATMENT

1. Use a vaporizer or humidifier at night. Even an old-fashioned tea kettle with a hot plate may be used. Direct the stream with a cone made of newspaper. If the child awakens with croupy coughing take him into the bathroom, close the windows and doors, and run hot water full-blast into the shower or tub to saturate the air with water vapor. It may be helpful to hold the child upright over your shoulder.
2. Avoid sudden temperature changes. Dress warmly at all times to prevent chilling, but guard against overheating.
3. Maintain good hydration with a good water intake. This will help loosen secretions. Avoid milk. Lukewarm liquids seem more effective than cold in decreasing respiratory distress. The extra fluid will help lubricate the bronchial passages. If a child is told to drink a small glass of water each time he coughs often after the third or fourth glass of water the cough will stop. Water is the very best cough medicine.

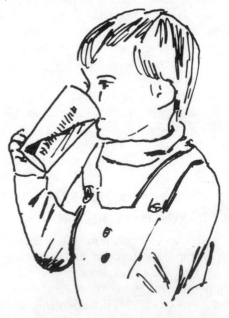

4. The child is often anxious and should not be left alone. Holding the child may be reassuring.
5. Fomentations to the neck and upper chest region may bring considerable relief. (92) Wring a bath towel out of hot water and place it between dry towels. More than one layer of towel may be necessary be-

tween the skin and the wet towel to prevent burning. Leave the towels in place until they begin cooling, then apply a fresh hot towel. After three or four applications wipe the area with a washcloth wrung from cold water, dry quickly, and cover the patient to prevent chilling. (See HOME REMEDIES for more detailed instructions.)

6. After the acute phase, a heating compress may be applied to the chest. Squeeze a thin piece of cotton fabric from cold water, place it against the chest, cover well on all sides with a piece of plastic, and hold in place with long strips of material such as bed sheeting, or a tight-fitting sweater.

7. Steroids (cortisone-like drugs) and antibiotics are of no value in viral croup, and may unnecessarily subject the child to the risk of an allergic or other adverse drug reaction. (90, 97)

8. Do not give cough syrup or other preparations for colds as these may inhibit the natural tendency to clear the throat by coughing or may dry and thicken secretions, making them more difficult to move.

9. Many cases of recurrent croup have been shown to be on an allergic basis. (94-96) A diet free of the common food allergens may be helpful. See Appendix B for the most common food allergens.

## DANDRUFF

Sebaceous or oil glands are found everywhere on the body surface except the palms and soles. The greatest number is found on the face and scalp. Sebum, the oily secretion, lubricates the hair and horny layer of the skin, to keep them soft and pliable. Sebum is an oily combination of water, fats, soaps, cholesterol and remains of dead cells that were once part of the gland. Underactive sebaceous glands cause dry hair and skin; overactive glands produce oily hair and skin. Sebum on the skin also serves to prevent the passage of water into or out of the skin. Excess sebum may collect to form dandruff. (119)

## TREATMENT

1. A number of shampoos are recommended for dandruff. Some of them contain antimicrobial agents to destroy scalp bacteria. It has not yet been demonstrated that antimicrobials have a beneficial effect on dandruff. (120, 121)

   Shampoos containing soap in any form cause itchiness and dandruff in sensitive individuals. A trial of 100 percent detergent shampoo is always worthwhile. Get a detergent such as Basic H or LOC (Shacklee or Amway, respectively – but not their shampoos which contain soap and fragrance), dilute about 20 times with water (l tablespoon to a cup, of water), and shampoo once or twice a week or more. Most people report improvement and many are cured.

Shampoos containing selenium sulfide have been shown to cause eye damage and hair loss. (122) We do not recommend their use.

2. The use of plain water shampoo, the detergent shampoo mentioned in 1, or a nonmedicated shampoo or soap every one to three days will remove dandruff flakes from the scalp as they form. (123)

3. Dipping cotton balls in a mouthwash such as Listerine and rubbing the scalp and hair with it is said to discourage dandruff. (124)

4. Cider vinegar has been reported useful in the treatment of dandruff. Warm the vinegar, pour it over the head, wrap the head in a towel for about an hour and then shampoo the hair. One lady reports that this treatment twice a week for a month cured her dandruff.

5. A combination of apple cider vinegar and castor oil may be tried. One person reports that he applied apple cider vinegar after a shower; after it dried, he rubbed castor oil vigorously into the scalp. One treatment was sufficient.

6. Aloe vera shampoo may be quite effective. It has a slight natural foaming action.

7. That diet may be a cause of dandruff is suggested in a 1957 article. (125) The authors felt that the large quantities of sugar and fat in the typical American diet cannot be absorbed by the body and may be the cause of extra scalp excretion. It is well known that sugar is temporarily stored in skin after a sugary meal.

8. For some people the use of biodegradable dish detergent as a shampoo may relieve the scalp itching. Rinse thoroughly. Dish detergent and ordinary shampoos are comparable in chemical composition. To be preferred, however, is the pure, soap-free detergent concentrate described in #1 above.

## DEPRESSION

Depression is a term frequently applied to a mood of gloom and sadness. Common symptoms are an appearance of sadness on the face, decreased energy, slowed thinking, movement without purpose or confidence, decreased appetite, perhaps with weight loss, sleep difficulties, and diminished sexual interest. The patient may report feeling irritable and fearful. In severe depression he may appear inefficient in his work, socially disorganized, and careless in his appearance.

Depression may be due to psychological or physiological problems. The loss of a loved one or a job are common causes. Situations which chronically thwart a sense of mastery and achievement over a period of time may precipitate depression. Circumstances that disrupt a person's sense of security, stability, effectiveness or worth generally provoke depression.

Patients with hepatitis or severe viral illness are prone to depression.

Alterations in the endocrine function such as Cushing's disease, Addison's disease, or the postpartum state are precipitants of depression. Stroke and certain other brain diseases may induce a prolonged depression. This type of depression may be due to some disturbed physiologic mechanisms in the central nervous system which are not yet understood.

Certain personality features seem to make some people more prone to depression than others. Insecure, sensitive, emotionally unstable, and immature people who tend to exaggerate emotional reactions of all types are apparently more prone to depression.

Certain people such as the slightly mentally retarded, who are limited in their ability to cope with difficulties are likely to develop depression.

## TREATMENT

1. It is the duty of everyone who professes to be a Christian to keep his thoughts under the control of reason and oblige himself to be cheerful and happy . . . Sadness deadens the circulation in the blood vessels and nerves, and also retards the action of the liver. It hinders the process of digestion and of nutrition, and has a tendency to dry up the marrow of the whole system . . . " (Reduce activity in the immune system) (127) "A merry heart doeth good like a medicine; but a broken spirit drieth the bones." (128)
2. Sage tea is said to help depression. (129) Catnip or alfalfa tea can be helpful. Use one cupful morning and night.
3. A deep breathing exercise should be carried out twice daily, as improper breathing causes gloom. (130) Take a deep breath, hold for a slow count of 20, exhale through the nose, and hold breath out for a count of 10. Repeat 30 to 50 times.
4. Meals should be on a regular schedule and nothing should be eaten between meals. Eating at irregular hours causes depression. (131)
5. A significant number of depressed persons have disordered circadian rhythms (biologic time clocks) and will greatly improve by simply going to bed two hours earlier. Sleep no more than nine hours daily.
6. Exercise studies have shown that depressed persons placed on a regular exercise program experience mood elevation. (132) Dr. Herbert DeVries, director of the University of Southern California's Exercise Physiology Laboratory states that exercise is more effective than tranquilizers in some cases of anxiety. A feeling of well-being and reduced tension is often associated with physical fitness.

   A variety of sports such as jogging, walking, and gardening have been shown effective. Purposeful outdoor exercise such as gardening is ideal, purposeless activity less so, and competitive sports least; for maximum psychological gains competition should be minimized. (133)

Although physical exercise on the job may be helpful, voluntary recreational programs have been shown more valuable.

7. Sunshine may be very beneficial in depression. Melatonin, a hormone produced by the body in darkness, causes depression. Light suppresses melatonin secretion. (134)

8. A strict weight reduction program frequently leads to depression and other mental symptoms. (135) Any weight reduction program should be gradual and should involve re-education in a lifestyle to be followed for the remainder of the life rather than a strict short-term "crash" diet.

9. Food allergy probably plays a far larger role in depression than has been hitherto recognized. Dr. William Crook, a prolific writer on allergies, observed that many of the symptoms of depression and food allergy are similar. (136) Other physicians have observed that removing refined carbohydrates from the diet of depressed people is often helpful. (137)

10. Approximately 200 drugs have been reported to cause depression. (138, 139) Chances are high that any medication used regularly or even occasionally is the cause of depression.

11. Caffeine has been found to induce depression. Groups of moderate and high caffeine users reported significantly higher depression scores when compared to non-users. (140, 142) The higher the total caffeine intake, the more likely the subjects were to suffer from depression. The researchers were unable to identify a clear-cut dosage level which produced symptoms.

12. Smokers report significantly higher levels of depression than do non-smokers. (142)

13. Low blood sugar (hypoglycemia) may induce depression. (143) Treat this disorder with exercise, regularity in all things, no more than three meals daily and ideally two (breakfast and lunch), a diet principally of fruits, vegetables and whole grains, and no sugar or free fats.

14. A high sugar diet may lead to depression. The B vitamins are known to be essential to mental health, and B vitamins are used up in the metabolism of sugar.

15. Antidepressant drugs have a number of adverse side effects. The major antidepressants may induce liver damage and hepatitis, jaundice (yellowing of the skin), dry mouth, constipation, blurred vision, sweating, rapid heart beat, delayed passage of urine, impotence, tremors, dizziness, fainting, muscular weakness, exaggeration of the reflexes, abnormal sensations, skin disorders, headache, insomnia, color blindness and behavioral changes, low blood pressure, abnormal blood conditions, irregular heart beat, and grand mal seizures. Minor antidepressants may cause cardiovascular irregularities, overactive reflexes, overstimulation, and a sense of euphoria. (144)

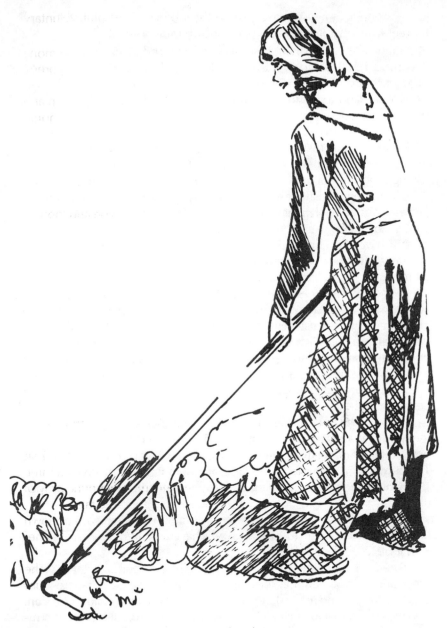

*Gardening is an excellent exercise to combat depression*

## DIABETES MELLITUS

Diabetes mellitus is currently the third largest killer in the United

States. About four to five percent of Americans develop diabetes mellitus. It is estimated that three-and-a-half to four million Americans have diabetes; about 40 percent of the cases are undiagnosed. (149) Approximately 200,000 to 300,000 new cases are diagnosed each year. The greatest number of diabetics are 45 years of age or older. Women are more likely to have it than men, and women over 45 who have had children have more diabetes.

Mellitus means "sweet" and comes from the fact that a blood glucose level above about 180 mg. percent causes excess sugar to spill over into the urine. (147) Diabetes comes from the Greek word meaning "to flow through" because of the large quantities of urine passed by diabetics.

Symptoms of diabetes include polydipsia (excessive thirst), polyuria (excessive urine), polyphagia (excessive eating), weight loss and lack of energy. Diabetics are usually prone to Candida (yeast) infections and may frequently have infections such as vulvitis (inflammation of the vulva) or balanitis (inflammation of the glans penis). Candida thrives on skin and mucous membranes storing large quantities of glucose.

Although it is rarely necessary to perform a glucose tolerance test, an abnormal blood sugar curve provides laboratory diagnosis of the disease. The blood sugar will rise higher and return to normal more slowly in a diabetic than in a non-diabetic. Usually only a single blood sugar level at two hours after a meal is ample evidence to make the diagnosis. Since glucose tolerance tests are stressful to the pancreas, they should be discouraged. A fasting blood sugar consistently above 120, and a two hour blood sugar persistently above 120 to 130 is usually diagnostic of diabetes.

Largely because of the prevalence of elevated blood sugar levels in the general population, the criteria for diagnosis of diabetes were revised upward rather drastically recently, a trend that we feel is most unfortunate. The new criteria prompted one diabetologist to remark, tongue-in-cheek, "Now our patients will be dying of carbohydrate intolerance rather than diabetes."

We find that a significant number of patients with high normal fasting blood sugars, in the 100 to 115 range, will have definitely abnormal curves with a glucose tolerance test.

There are two types of diabetes: juvenile-and adult-onset. However, age alone is not a criterion for diagnosis, since "juvenile" diabetes may occur at any age and the "adult-onset" type may occur in children. Recent studies suggest that juvenile diabetes may be the result of a viral infection such as mumps, German measles, flu, or infectious mononucleosis. It is felt that the virus remains in the body, and invades and destroys the beta cells (insulin-producing cells in the pancreas) in susceptible persons. Juvenile diabetes generally appears while the person is young. Onset may be sudden. Symptoms of diabetes in children are for the most part the same as in adults. The child, however, is more likely to be underweight than overweight. The juvenile diabetic will not respond to oral hypoglycemic drugs and must be given insulin. Juvenile diabetics may be brought to medical attention because of growth failure despite a huge appetite. Growth of diabetic children appears to be related to the degree of control of the diabetes. Many juvenile diabetics approximate adult height after prolonged growth periods, but the onset of diabetes just prior to a growth period may interfere with achieving full adult height.

The course of juvenile diabetes is often unstable and blood sugar levels vary between being too high and too low. Control is often difficult and is referred to as "brittle."

Because insulin requirements are based on body size, the child will require more insulin as he grows. This often causes the patient and his parents to feel that the condition is worsening. The juvenile diabetic should be under the care of a specialist, at least initially, since life expectancy may be drastically reduced without meticulous control. The patient and family should be thoroughly conversant with his disease, its complications, and ideal treatment in his particular case. We believe that every diabetic on insulin should have and use regularly one of the inexpensive instruments to measure blood sugars rapidly (one to two minutes) with a fingerstick.

Juvenile-onset diabetes may also be called insulin-dependent or Type I diabetes.

Adult-onset (maturity onset, non-insulin dependent, or Type II) diabetes generally occurs in persons over 40 years of age. The patient is typically overweight and presents with one or two mild symptoms. Susceptibility to diabetes may be increased by a combination of obesity and inactivity. (149) These patients are able to produce part of their own insulin. About 80 percent of overweight adults develop diabetes.

Because in simple obesity there is insulin resistance, treatment of maturity onset diabetes is aimed at achieving ideal body weight while maintaining adequate nutritional status. Once overweight is corrected the patient almost always requires less or even no administered insulin. Because insulin requirements are based on body size it is well for the diabetic to be slightly leaner than his ideal body weight by five to ten percent.

Coronary heart disease and disease of the small and large blood vessels are much more common in the diabetic than in the non-diabetic. Almost 75 percent of the diabetic deaths in the United States are due to vascular disease.

Oral antidiabetic medications are not insulin. There is currently much debate about their safety. One study revealed a higher death rate from cardiovascular disease in patients given oral antidiabetics than in diabetics given insulin. (148)

Diabetics taking Diabinese, Orinase, and Dymelor, as well as other oral antidiabetic drugs may develop severe anemia, jaundice, or hypoglycemic coma. In one study, patients complaining of shortness of breath, dizziness, and feeling bad showed very low hemoglobin, hematocrit, reticuloycte and red blood cell counts due to pure red blood cell aplasia (failure of formation in the bone marrow). (170, 171)

Diabetes may develop secondary to other diseases such as cirrhosis of the liver, pancreatitis, tumor or cystic fibrosis of the pancreas, and disorders of the pituitary, adrenals, or thyroid. (149)

The pancreas, a long gland that lies immediately behind the stomach is composed of two types of tissue: acinar and islets of Langerhans. The acini secrete digestive juices into the intestines. The islets of Langerhans secrete hormones which go directly into the blood.

The islets of Langerhans are made up of two different types of cells, alpha and beta. The alpha cells secrete glucagon, a substance which stimulates the conversion of glycogen to glucose, raising the blood glucose level; while the beta cells secrete insulin, preventing the sugar level from going too high.

The basic function of insulin is to increase the rate of glucose transport through the cellular membrane. The membrane pores are too small to allow the glucose molecule to gain entrance to the cell by the process of simple diffusion, so glucose must be carried through the membrane combined with a chemical carrier. Without insulin only a small amount of glucose can combine with the carrier and be transported into the cells. With normal amounts of insulin the transfer is increased three to five times, and with large amounts of insulin the glucose transfer may be increased 15 to 25-fold. The cells of the brain, intestine, renal tubules, and red blood cells are able to absorb glucose without insulin because they use a different transport mechanism.

Insulin enhances those reactions that lower the blood glucose level and inhibits those that raise it. Most other metabolic hormones have the opposite effect – they act to increase the blood glucose level.

Glucagon's action in the liver is opposite to insulin's. Glucagon acts mainly on the liver. It is quickly deactivated and reaches the general circulation in only minute amounts. Glucagon increases the formation of glucose by the breakdown of glycogen and fat breakdown (gluconeogenesis) increasing also the fatty acid supply.

Glucagon secretion depends on the blood glucose level; glucagon secretion is increased by low blood sugar and decreased by high blood sugar. (46) This balance maintains blood sugar within normal limits.

Diabetes mellitus results from failure of the pancreas to produce insulin, increased and unmet insulin requirements, or an excess of insulin antagonists. It is caused by degeneration of the beta cells of the islets of Langerhans in the pancreas. Hereditary appears to be a strong predisposing factor, especially in the adult-onset diabetic. The disease occurs at a progressively earlier age with each generation of diabetics. (149) Persons with a family history of diabetes should be encouraged to maintain their weight slightly below the ideal levels throughout their lifetime due to the association of diabetes and obesity.

Failure to utilize sufficient quantities of glucose for energy is the primary abnormality in diabetes. Because of this the blood glucose level rises often two to three times normal. The kidney tubules cannot reabsorb all the glucose that enters them, so large quantities of glucose are lost in the urine. Osmotic pressure in the tubules produced by the excess tubular glucose diminishes the reabsorption of water and the diabetic loses large amounts of both water and glucose in the urine. This, in turn, leads to polydipsia, or increased or excessive thirst, and even finally to dehydration.

Since the diabetic cannot utilize glucose for energy he loses weight and is weakened by excess consumption of his protein and fat stores. Because of this nutrient deficiency the diabetic may become very hungry and eat voraciously. (145) The excessive food intake common in diabetics is called polyphagia.

In the absence of adequate glucose the major share of energy is provided by fats. Large deposits of fats are broken down, releasing free fatty acids and ketone bodies, products of fatty acid metabolism, into the blood. These bodies dissociate, releasing hydrogen ions into the body fluids. The pH falls, causing the blood to become progessively more acid, with a decrease in plasma bicarbonate and increasing the $pCO2$ level in the arterial blood. This condition is called ketoacidosis, and may rapidly become life-threatening. Fortunately, it rarely occurs except in some juvenile diabetics.

Our treatment section is directed primarily toward the adult-onset, non-insulin dependent type. However, many of the principles will also apply to the juvenile diabetic.

## TREATMENT

1. We have observed excellent response in many diabetics to the Health Recovery Program. (See Appendix A)
2. There is evidence that a fiber-depleted diet may lead to diabetes. (150) High fiber diets have been shown to lower blood sugar levels after meals, decrease insulin requirements, and increase tissue sensitivity to insulin. Unrefined natural foods should be used in place of the low fiber, highly refined carbohydrates. A number of researchers have observed populations who were previously isolated from refined, processed foods, experiencing a striking increase in diabetes when exposed to refined carbohydrates. (151)
3. Overeating, particularly when combined with obesity and inactivity is felt to be associated with the rising incidence of maturity-onset diabetes. (152)
4. A diet high in complex carbohydrates and leguminous fiber has been shown to improve diabetic control. (156) A diet high in complex car-

bohydrates results in lower insulin requirements. (157) Apparently fibers delay the absorption of carbohydrates and produce a less marked rise in glucose levels after meals. (158) A group of volunteers given eight different varieties of dried beans demonstrated a mean peak rise in blood glucose levels at least 45 percent lower than a similar group of volunteers given 24 other common foods. (159) Dr. Holbrooke S. Seltzer of the University of Texas Southwestern Medical School in Dallas reports that a diet of complex carbohydrates is broken down more slowly than simple sugars, allowing more efficient use of the insulin produced by the body. (60)

5. Green beans and onions appear to lower blood sugar according to a West German study. A diet of 68 percent carbohydrates, 20 percent fat, and 12 percent protein was given to a group of diabetics. On this diet, fasting blood sugar levels and those two hours after eating averaged 227.98 mg/ 100 ml. The same diet with the addition of green beans produced blood sugar levels averaging only 194.9 mg/100 ml. Fresh onions produced a significant reduction in the blood sugar level of a group of outpatient diabetics. (162)

6. A diet high in raw foods may be quite helpful in controlling blood sugar. One patient had his insulin requirements reduced from 60 to 15 units per day merely by increasing the percentage of raw foods in the diet. The authors of the study recommend that fruits and melons not be eaten in large quantities. (163) A 1982 study revealed that the blood glucose response to apples and bananas was almost identical to the response to pure glucose. (164)

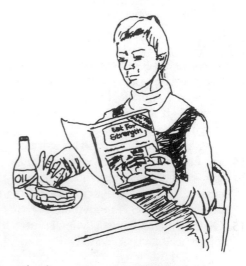

*Eliminating fats from the diet can lower the blood sugar levels*

7. Milk and sugar combinations may play a major role in diabetes production. Both lead to obesity and lowered resistance to infection, two factors shown to be pertinent to the pathogenesis of diabetes mellitus. (165)

8. Coffee may induce extraordinarily high blood sugar levels. (167) Diabetics should avoid all substances containing caffeine. Six hours after having been given caffeine "diabetic rats" demonstrated blood sugar levels that were twice usual. Normal rats, however, given caffeine showed an opposite effect – caffeine caused their blood sugar levels to fall by half within 12 hours after administration.

9. The nitrate/nitrites used in meat curing may be a cause of diabetes. Physicians in Iceland noticed that the consumption of chemically cured/smoked mutton is unusually high during the Christmas-New Year season, and that there is an abnormally high number of diabetics born in October – nine months after the feast. (168)

10. Sixty diabetics given a fat-free diet demonstrated a decrease in the blood sugar level and in the amount of sugar spilled in the urine. The drop occurred rapidly, on the first or second day of the fat-free diet.

11. When and how a diabetic eats is fully as important as what he eats. Regular meals train the pancreas to perform on a regular schedule and allow rest periods to assist in its recovery.

Hasty eating does not result in the most favorable blood sugar levels. It was found that in patients with shorter eating times there was greater glucose instability, that is, the fluctuations were greater in fast eaters. Hasty eaters also showed a fluctuation in body weight. A part of the treatment of every patient with diabetes should be instruction on how to eat slowly to obtain the best possible blood sugar level. (166)

12. Ten gm. of raw garlic per day lead to a reduction in the amount of sugar spilled in the urine in one study. (161)

13. Certain drugs such as corticosteroids and thiazide diuretics may cause diabetes. (152) Oral contraceptives may make blood sugar control difficult. (153) Nicotinic acid (a B vitamin) is suspected of inducing diabetes when given in large doses. Approximately 12 percent of patients given benzothiadiazine-containing drugs develop diabetes. (155)

14. Because diabetics are unusually prone to infection, and often have slow healing they should do all they can to maintain an optimal level of health. A consistent daily routine with adequate rest and sleep will be of great value in this.

15. Foot care is very important in diabetics. The following suggestions may be helpful:
   A. Wash the feet daily with mild soap and lukewarm water. Dry carefully, particularly between the toes.
   B. Check daily for cuts, scratches and blisters.

C. Wear comfortable, properly fitted shoes and socks. Socks should be of an absorbent material such as cotton.
D. Keep the feet warm at all times. Cold feet will have a decreased supply of blood, which may encourage infection.
E. Avoid garters and stockings with seams as they hinder blood flow.
F. Don't wear thongs between the toes.
G. Do not cut or use chemical agents on calluses or corns. Have your physician or podiatrist care for them.
H. Avoid pointed or open-toe shoes and high heels. Shoes should not squeeze the toes. Changing shoes during the day helps prevent perspiration.
I. Don't walk barefooted. Wear sneakers or sandals at the beach. Rubber or vinyl does not allow evaporation of perspiration and should not be worn frequently or for long periods.
J. Hot water bottles or heating pads should not be used if there is decreased sensation in the feet as they may cause burning. Test water temperature before bathing.
K. A small amount of moisturizing lotion may be used to soften dry skin on the heels and soles. Solid vegetable shortening is effective and inexpensive. (172) Do not apply between the toes or around the toenails.
L. Avoid medicated powders. For sweating feet use cornstarch or unscented talc.

16. Do not smoke. Nicotine constricts blood vessels, which reduces blood flow. (175) Smokers have higher insulin requirements than do non-smokers. (176) Heavy smokers may require 30 percent more insulin than non-smokers. (177)

17. Many medications enhance the effect of diabetic drugs. (175) Even over-the-counter medications should be taken only under the supervision of a physician. Many antacids contain sugar although it is not listed on the table of ingredients. (178) This unsuspected source of sugar may make diabetes control very difficult.

18. Regular exercise is extremely beneficial to diabetics. Physical fitness improves glucose tolerance and may retard the cardiovascular complications which accompany diabetes. (179) During acute exercise insulin levels fall, stimulating glucose production by the liver. Exercise also increases body sensitivity to insulin and changes insulin binding to receptors. Insulin binding is proportional to the level of physical fitness. (180,181) The overweight, sedentary diabetic often has markedly decreased insulin binding, which means that the insulin he is producing is relatively ineffective. Fortunately, exercise and weight reduction can significantly enhance insulin binding and effectiveness.

19. Fasting for one to five days may be very useful in the obese adult-onset diabetic. Under medical supervision, fasting (with insulin omitted) has

been found to markedly decrease or eliminate insulin requirements in the overweight adult-onset diabetic (see NUTRITION FOR VEGETAR-IANS for more complete description.)

PLEASE NOTE: The fasting, in selected cases, is done *only* under medical supervision. As a general rule, the juvenile diabetic should *never* fast.

## ECZEMA

Eczema is a term loosely applied to a variety of skin diseases. It is generally characterized in the early stages by redness, weeping, oozing, and crusting, and later by scaling, thickening, and pigmentation of the skin. There may be small blister-like lesions. The word "eczema" comes from a Greek word meaning "the result of boiling over or out."

Infantile eczema is fairly common. It usually appears between two months and two years of age. It is the commonest and earliest manifestation of allergy. Many of these children will later develop asthma or hay fever. They often have a family history of allergy.

## TREATMENT

1. Aloe vera gel may be applied to the inflamed area. (182)
2. Oatmeal baths may be quite soothing. See the section on chickenpox for procedure.
3. Avoid contact with wool, nylon, suede, and other common contact irritants. Man-made fibers should be avoided. Silk or cotton should be worn next to the skin.
4. Severe flareups can often be aborted by using artificial fever therapy. (See HOME REMEDIES for procedure.)
5. Some drugs induce eczema. One woman on birth control pills developed widespread eczema which continued to worsen despite treatment until the pills were stopped. (183) Even when drugs do not initiate the eczema, they often worsen or prolong the course.
6. Alkaline or soda baths have been used successfully in eczema. Add one cup of baking soda to a tub of water at approximately 94 to 98 degrees. The patient should sit in the tub, dipping water up on the body parts not covered by the water. After 30 to 60 minutes in the tub the patient should stand in the tub to allow water to drip off. Blot the skin dry with a towel rather than rubbing it. Do not get chilled.
7. Soap may be irritating and should be used sparingly if at all. Soap need not be used except on hands and feet, as the rest of the body can be properly cleansed by water alone. Detergents, perfumes, and other chemicals should not be allowed in contact with the skin.
8. A trial period of eliminating the most common food allergens may be very beneficial. See Appendix B for a list of the foods. After a week without any of the foods on the list a single food may be added back

to the diet every three to five days. Any response during the time suggests sensitivity and the food should be eliminated from the diet. Most common offenders are milk, eggs, chocolate, citrus and wheat. Strict avoidance of all dairy products for three to four weeks should be tried in all cases. Since tiny amounts of milk protein may cause trouble in the sensitive person, read labels; dried milk powder is found in most baked goods.

9. If skin is dry and crusted, oil may be applied with a soft cloth.

10. A bath with two cups of cornstarch in the water may be effective in relieving itching. (184)

11. Avoid temperature extremes or rapid temperature changes. Keep the skin warm at all times. The body's own healing mechanisms are more active at body temperature.

12. Protect from infection. Contact with herpes simplex virus, fresh vaccine lesions, etc. should be avoided. Use caution with routine immunizations, as flareups are possible.

13. Do not scratch the lesions. A "vaseline milk" may soothe itching and encourage healing. Immediately after washing and while the skin is still wet, rub a bit of vaseline into the water clinging to the hands. This forms a milky fluid which should be gently smoothed onto the affected skin and allowed to dry. Do not rub skin across skin lines, but in the direction of skin lines (around arms and legs rather than up and down). Even rubbing (to say nothing of scratching) can cause microscopic cracks in the skin to worsen eczema.

14. Red clover and golden seal tea may be used as a cold compress to skin lesions for 20 minutes four times a day. The astringent action (pulling skin together) is the healing feature. The tea may be drunk also. Comfrey tea may be applied as a compress but should not be drunk as it is suspected to increase cancer risk in the esophagus.

15. Many researchers feel that eczema may be prevented by breast-feeding infants for at least four months. A 1981 study revealed that children with allergic parents given solid food within four months after birth had over two and a half times the rate of eczema of children who had non-allergic parents and who were not given solid food within four months. The rate of eczema increased in almost direct proportion to the number of different kinds of solid foods eaten. (185)

16. Several studies have shown that breast-fed children can develop eczema from foods eaten by the mother. Eggs, milk, and soybeans eaten by breastfeeding mothers have all been shown to produce eczema in their infants. (185, 186)

17. Sunlight is beneficial in most patients; in a few, sunlight worsens the condition. Avoid any degree of sunburning.

18. Many eczema patients have impaired glucose tolerance levels. (187) The Health Recovery Program (Appendix A) may be quite helpful.

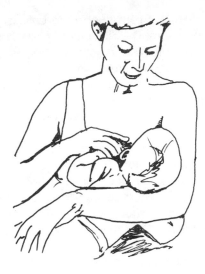

19. Charcoal baths may be quite useful. Put one-half to one cup of pow-
    dered charcoal in a tub of lukewarm water. Soak once or twice daily
    for thirty minutes. Finish with a tepid shower (no soap!) to remove
    charcoal and pat dry.
20. Evening primrose oil, applied to the inflamed skin areas after one of
    the soothing baths mentioned above, has been reported to be very ef-
    fective. It may also be taken internally. The primrose oil is a rich source
    of gamma linolenic acid, an essential fatty acid which is the precursor
    of certain prostaglandins; these are very potent hormones produced
    in the body. They are antiinflammatory and improve the body's de-
    fense mechanisms. *The oil is not a substitute for identification and
    elimination of offending allergens.*

## EMPHYSEMA

Emphysema is a disease resulting from coughing and wheezing,
caused most often by smoking. It is one of the fastest growing diseases in
the modern world. Part of the increase is due to the fact that people are
living longer, but smoking and air pollution are the main factors in the rise
of emphysema cases. It is the most common chronic lung condition and
the major cause of pulmonary dysfunction. It has been estimated that
more than 10 million Americas have emphysema, and more than twice
that number have lung conditions bordering on emphysema.

Emphysema is generally first diagnosed between the ages of 55 and
65. It is approximately nine times as common in men as in women, perhaps due to the difference in smoking habits and exposure to air pollutants. The name "emphysema" comes from a Greek word meaning "to
puff up with air."

Shortness of breath due to the collapse of the airways is the most common symptom. The difficulty is greatest on exhaling, or breathing out. The neck veins often stand out from the effort, and the patient commonly purses the lips and breathes through the mouth to help keep the air passages open. Wheezing may be present on expiration. Breathing in is generally rapid and short. The patient may breathe 25 to 30 times a minute and still receive an inadequate supply of air. People with long-term emphysema often develop clubbing or enlargement of the end of the fingers. Sometimes patients with emphysema are referred to as "pink puffers" because of the ruddy color which the face may take on. Over a period of time the patient develops a barrel-shaped chest which is very characteristic of emphysema. The chest appears to be overinflated. The emphysema patient often speaks in short, jerky phrases and commonly appears gaunt and anxious. Minor activity may produce extreme shortness of breath and exhaustion.

The human body requires a great deal of oxygen. The average grown man takes in about a pint of air with each breath. If he breathes about 14 times a minute he takes in about seven quarts of air each minute. The lungs take in about 600 to 1,000 cubic feet of air each day. You require about a square yard of lung space for each 2 1/5 pounds of body weight. A grown man needs lung space about as large as a tennis court. It would seem impossible to get this much lung space inside the human chest, but our Creator made provision for all our needs. The trachea, or windpipe, branches off into two divisions called bronchi. In the lung the bronchi divide into smaller branches which then branch off into the even smaller bronchioles. These bronchioles end in hundreds of millions of little air sacs called alveoli. The walls of alveoli are extremely thin, consisting of a single layer of cells only 0.0004 inch thick. The average alveolus is only 250 microns in diameter; forty of them placed side-by-side would measure only 2/5 of an inch! (192)

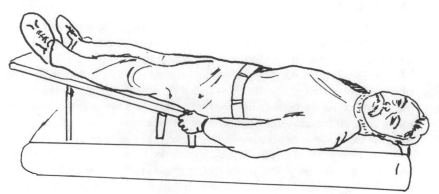

*Postural drainage*

In emphysema a large portion of the walls of the alveoli (terminal air sacs in the lungs) are destroyed. The surface area of the pulmonary membrane becomes reduced, sometimes to less than one-fourth of the normal value. Aeration of the blood is diminished as a result of these losses.

## TREATMENT:

1. If the emphysema patient continues to smoke all treatment is ineffective. Studies show a relationship between smoking and decreased ability to force air out of the lungs. The average heavy smoker has only half the ability to force air out of his lungs as a nonsmoker. Cough and sputum production are and sputum production are often improved when the patient stops smoking.

2. Exercise trains skeletal muscles to function more efficiently and should be part of the daily program of every emphysema patient. Breathing exercises are often helpful:

   A. The patient should blow his nose to clear the air passages at the start. Patient should attempt to make this type of breathing habitual.

   B. The patient sits in a straight chair, with legs spread apart and feet flat on the floor. Placing a small pillow firmly against his abdomen, he should bend forward over it, breathing out slowly through pursed lips as if blowing out a candle.

   C. The patient lies on the floor on his back and raises his head, shoulders and arms to reach below his knees. He should simultaneously contract the muscles of the abdomen, breathing out until he feels the urge to breathe in again. As he relaxes back to the horizontal position he should breathe out slowly.

   The purpose of these exercises is to train the patient to breathe with his abdominal muscles rather than with the upper thorax. Thoracic breathing is common in emphysema patients and in women who have changed their breathing habits because of the constricting effects of girdles and corsets. Exercises may induce wheezing and coughing, but the patient should be assured that this is expected.

3. The patient should be instructed that slow, deep breathing relieves shortness of breath more quickly than rapid and shallow breaths.

4. Inhaled irritants, narcotics, sedatives and unnecessary surgery may all aggravate the symptoms of emphysema. (194)

5. Patients living at high atmosphere (above 4000 feet) may be benefited by a move to lower altitude.

6. The chances of a male between the ages of 50 and 70 dying of a lung disease such as bronchitis or emphysema is twice as great if he lives in an area with a high level of air pollution. (195) Persons living in these

areas may profit by a move to a less polluted area. Avoid outdoor activities when air pollution levels are high.

7. Keep the living area as dust-free as possible. Air filters may be used to remove pollutants and particles from the air. A room humidifier used during winter months may allow dust particles to settle. (196) Avoid cigarette smoke, pollens, fumes, and aerosols. Avoid dusting and sweeping. Keep the kitchen well ventilated.

8. Use a warming scarf or mask over the mouth and nose when outdoors in cold weather. Keep the body warm at all times.

9. The fluid intake should be kept high to keep sputum thin and easy to raise.

10. Nebulized water inhalations may be given to humidify the bronchial tree and thin sputum.

11. The patient should be taught an exercise called "controlled coughing" in which he inhales slowly and deeply, exhales through pursed lips, and coughs in short "huffing" bursts rather than vigorously.

12. Emphysema patients should avoid contact with individuals who have any type of respiratory tract infection.

13. Postural drainage exercises should be carried out daily. Each position should be utilized for 5 to 15 minutes. Postural drainage may be performed by lying on a tilt table or bed with the foot elevated 18 inches. The patient lies on his back, right side, left side, and stomach to allow clearing of all segments of the lungs.

14. Avoid drugs which suppress cough and dry up secretions.

15. Excessively hot or cold foods may induce coughing and should be avoided.

16. Hard-to-chew foods tire the patient and should be avoided. Gas forming foods cause distention, restricting movement of the diaphragm. Never overeat. Use a low salt diet.

17. Do not eat when emotionally upset or angry.

18. The patient should be given a low-calorie diet designed to maintain optimal weight. Generally, the thinner the patient the smaller the amount of flesh that must be supplied with oxygen and nutrients. Obesity and constipation decrease the patient's resistance to respiratory infection. (197)

19. Three, four, or five inch blocks under the foot of the bed will help prevent mucus from accumulating in the lower part of the lungs during the night.

## ENDOMETRIOSIS

Endometriosis is a condition in which tissues which resemble the lining of the uterus, or womb, occur in other places. Tissue implants may be found in the ovary, ligaments, bladder, rectum, bowel, appendix, and other sites. These tissues respond to the same hormonal influences that induce menstruation, and bleed at the time of the menstrual period.

There are two types of endometriosis: true endometriosis is also called external endometriosis. In this type the tissue implants are found outside the uterine wall. In internal endometriosis, also called adenomyosis, the growths are inside the uterine wall.

The cause of endometriosis is still unknown but probably the most commonly accepted theory is that during menstruation some menstrual products back up through the fallopian tubes onto the ovaries or other areas of the pelvic cavity, particularly during sexual excitation.

Symptoms of endometriosis include pain with menstruation, inability to become pregnant, and abnormal vaginal bleeding. Many women with endometriosis do not even know they have it until they see a physician because they are unable to be become pregnant. The pain of endometriosis generally begins prior to the menstrual period, lasts through the period, and sometimes for a couple of days afterward. It is usually at its worst just prior to the onset of bleeding and for the first day or two of the period. Most patients are between 30 and 40 years of age at the time of diagnosis. Symptoms often begin to appear in the early twenties.

A 1983 report tells of neurological problems associated with endometriosis, and cautions doctors to consider endometriosis as a possible cause of low-back and lower extremity pain in women. One 28-year-old woman had right foot drop each month prior to her period which disappeared 48 hours after it. She had had the symptoms for four years at the time the authors of the report examined her. The second case was a 38-year-old woman with severe pain in the lower back which radiated down the legs. In both cases the physicians observed implants of endometrial tissue on the lumbosacral plexus. (198)

Approximately 25 to 30% of white women suffer from endometriosis, but it is relatively rare in black women. There may be some tendency for endometriosis to run in families.

Interestingly, becoming pregnant seems to slow down progression of the disease, and this slowing effect continues during the period of lactation. However, the protective effect of pregnancy and lactation does not always occur, and when it does it is not a permanent cure. Endometriosis has a tendency to continue to worsen as long as the woman menstruates, but after menopause it becomes inactive, although scar tissue remains.

## TREATMENT

1. Many physicians have in the past used oral contraceptives (birth control pills) in the treatment of endometriosis but we now know that they actually stimulate endometriosis by stimulating the receptor sites of these implants, causing growth. (199)
2. Internal fetal monitoring has now been linked to future development of

endometriosis. A study done at the University of Wisconsin revealed that 24% of women with internal monitors developed endometriosis, while only 8 percent without monitors later developed endometriosis. (200)

3. Avoiding sexual activity during the menstrual period may lessen the risk of developing endometriosis. After orgasm there is a negative intrauterine pressure that may induce a suction mechanism. (201)

4. Because endometriosis tends to subside after menopause many women choose to use no treatment and to merely wait until they "outgrow" the symptoms.

5. A diet high in plant steroids may be quite helpful in endometriosis. This diet includes apples, cherries, olives, plums, wheat germ, all whole grains except millet, carrots, peanuts, all dried beans and peas, yams, bell pepper, eggplant, potatoes, tomatoes, parsley, sage, clover, alfalfa leaf tea, licorice root tea, red raspberry leaf tea, food yeast, garlic, anise seed, coconut, and all nuts.

6. Alternating hot and cold sitz baths for 20 to 30 minutes may be useful in reducing congestion of the pelvic organs, as may a hot foot bath for 30 minutes. Finish off either treatment with a cold mitten friction. Hot fomentations to the lower abdomen are very useful, and when carried out faithfully have resulted in a complete remission of symptoms. One of our patients, almost totally disabled from pain, had progressive improvement and final complete clearing of symptoms after fomentations for one year.

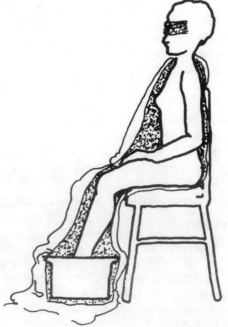

7. Some people obtain relief from the use of either an ice bag or a hot water bottle or heating pad on the lower abdomen or back.
8. Alfalfa or red raspberry leaf tea may be used.
9. Some women report relief of symptoms with a stretching exercise. Measure a line on the floor two feet from a wall. Stand with the tips of the toes on the line, and keeping the heels flat on the floor, lean the whole body toward the wall, hands at about shoulder height. When the chest touches the wall hold the position for ten seconds, push back into the upright position for five seconds, then repeat the exercise three times. Turn to the side, putting the right outer edge of the foot on the line, and lean sideways toward the wall, attempting to touch the hip to the wall. Hold for ten seconds and repeat. Do the same procedure with the left hip. Do the exercises three times a day for three days, then once a day for thirty days.

## FATIGUE

Tiredness is a common complaint in America today. With the labor-saving devices found all about us one would think that fatigue would never be a problem, but the opposite is true – fatigue is a more common complaint today than it was 100 years ago.

Fatigue is more likely a consequence of underexertion than it is of overexertion. Increased physical activity is often the treatment of choice for tiredness.

The causes of fatigue may be divided into two general classes: physiological and psychological. Psychological causes include such factors as depression, boredom, stress, and anxiety.

Physiological causes of fatigue are many and include bacterial or influenzal infections, heart disease, endocrine disorders, anemia, malnutrition, cancer, neurological disorders such as Parkinson's disease, multiple sclerosis, postconcussion syndrome, medications, arthritis, rheumatism, emphysema, hepatitis, undulant fever, infectious mononucleosis, tuberculosis and diabetes.

Physiological fatigue worsens as the day progresses, while psychological fatigue is generally present upon awakening in the morning.

## TREATMENT

1. Dehydration is often the cause of fatigue. A lack of water reduces work performance more rapidly than a lack of food. Thirst is not an adequate guide to the water requirements of man. Dehydration may exist without any awareness on the part of the individual.
2. Physical activity is a very effective treatment for fatigue. Rest is not a solution for fatigue in many cases, as tiredness is often the result of poor physical conditioning. Poor circulation decreases the ability of the body to eliminate the toxic products of metabolism. Inactivity is the

real basis of fatigue – think how tired you often are on Monday morning after a weekend of "rest." People who exercise regularly need less
oxygen to perform the same amount of work as a man who spends his
life in inactivity.

3. Indoor living may lead to fatigue because of an inadequate supply of
   fresh air. Daily out-of-doors exercise is the first step in the treatment of
   fatigue.

4. Overeating is a tax upon the body and may induce fatigue. Eat enough
   to satisfy hunger but not necessarily appetite. The act of metabolizing
   extra food is an unnecessary tax upon the body energies. Stomach
   stretching caused by overeating may interfere with the function of the
   diaphragm and makes breathing more difficult, diminishing the supply
   of oxygen available to the body. (211)

5. Many drugs are known to induce fatigue, including amphetamines,
   depressants, diuretics and some blood pressure medications. Many
   other drugs probably induce fatigue. (202, 203)

6. Fatigue is known to be a symptom of allergy. (204) A trial of a diet free
   of the most common food allergens may be quite helpful. See Appendix B for a list of these foods.

7. A group of 30 children seen at an air force hospital with complaints of
   fatigue were given a most unusual prescription. The doctors ordered
   that the children not watch any television at all. The symptoms van-
   ished within two to three weeks in every child who was kept strictly on
   the program. Those who continued to watch television but on a more
   limited basis had a reduction in symptoms, but not a complete remission. (205)

8. People who are compulsive often complain of continuous fatigue.
   They feel that they cannot relax until everything that needs to be done
   is finished. They cannot stop until everything on their list is complete,
   despite the fact that they are weary.

9. Improper diet induces many cases of fatigue. Using refined foods, full
   of artificial colorings and additives, high in sugars and fats does not
   supply the body with the "premium" fuel which will enable the body
   to function at its peak level.

10. Ideal blood sugar levels are important to energy levels. Both high and
    low blood sugar levels may lead to fatigue. An inadequate breakfast
    may result in a mid-morning drop in blood sugar levels. The use of
    sugar-laden snack foods may provide a temporary lift, but the low that
    follows is worse than before the sugar was consumed.

11. Low blood pressure may cause feelings of fatigue. Outdoor exercise is
    the best treatment for low blood pressure along with drinking lots of
    water. Low blood pressure often results from chronic dehydration.
    Use lots of fruits and vegetables, and few heavy, rich, or concentrated
    foods.

12. Insecticides and radioactivity are reported to cause fatigue. (206)
13. Fluorides, lead, mercury, cadmium and copper may cause fatigue. (207)
14. Boredom can drain your energies and make you chronically tired. Take up a new hobby, go to work a new way, do something out of the ordinary to relieve boredom. Half an hour of acute boredom can use more nervous energy than you expend in a whole days' work.
15. People whose work is primarily mental often become more fatigued than those with work of a physical nature. Only four hours' sleep is required to restore physical energy, but it may require twice that long to restore mental energy. To do mental work with a minimum of fatigue be certain that there is an adequate supply of fresh air to insure that the brain receives sufficient oxygen.
16. A diet high in sugar may induce fatigue. (208)
17. Being overweight puts an extra load on the circulatory and muscular systems of the body and hastens fatigue. The letters f-a-t are the first three letters in the word "fatigue." Isaac Stern, a violinist, says "Everyone knows that a fat man usually is a tired man." (209) Carrying around a lot of extra weight is certain to make one tired.
18. Too much protein, especially protein of animal origin, may make a person tired. Meat contains urinary or fatigue wastes in it. A pound of beef may contain fourteen grains of uric acid, a urinary waste. These waste products are not found in proteins of vegetable origin. (210)
19. Coffee, vitamin supplements, alcohol and sleeping pills are at best only a temporary solution, and at the worst are counterproductive. Excessive use of coffee and other caffeine-containing beverages is a prominent cause of fatigue.
20. Depression and fatigue are commonly seen together. One writer estimates that 85% of all patients seen in private medical practices show signs of mild depression with easy fatigability. See the section on depression for treatment suggestions. (211)
21. Stress and fatigue have much in common and are often observed in the same individual. Remember that exercise neutralizes stress.
22. Regularity in eating habits helps the body to adjust to a pattern of rest and work which allows it to conserve its energies. Regularity in sleeping is also essential.
23. Many people complaining of fatigue need to overcome habits of hurry or of sluggishness or indolence. Many people overreact to life situations, and expend energy needed for other activities. (211)
24. Vitamin, mineral or protein deficiency caused by many of the fad diets used for weight reduction deplete energy, inducing fatigue. Any weight reduction program should be sensible and well balanced.
25. Henry Ford, Sr. stated that a day of rest is essential. "We would have had our Model A car in production six months sooner, if I had forbid-

den my engineers to work on Sunday," Ford said. "It took us all week
to straighten out the mistakes they made on the day when they should
have rested." (209)
26. Loud noises are fatiguing. A group of researchers at Bellevue Hospital
    in New York popped an inflated paper bag near the head of a group
    of patients. Brain pressure increased to four times normal whether the
    patient expected the noise or not. A second noise a few seconds later
    induced even greater increases in brain pressure. Noise may induce fa-
    tigue without the subject being aware of it. Both quality and quantity
    of work suffer under noisy conditions.
27. Cigarette smoke made a group of laboratory rats two-thirds less active
    than a group of rats not exposed to smoke. The "smoking" rats spent
    their time lying limply, while the "non-smoking" rats ran and frolicked
    on a treadmill. A brisk walk out of doors is a better source of refresh-
    ment than a cigarette and cup of coffee. Coffee has adverse effects on
    blood sugar levels and leads to fatigue.
28. The physical environment may contribute to fatigue. Cluttered and
    messy working quarters and lack of elbow room may be more tiring
    than overwork. White colors are fatiguing, as are purple, brown, or-
    ange and even some shades of blue. Medium green and yellow are
    restful colors. Glare of glass and metal tables may induce fatigue. (209)

## FEVER BLISTERS

Fever blisters, or cold sores, are caused by herpes viruses. The virus
is transmitted by air and by direct contact.

Early symptoms are tingling, burning, and itching in the area of infection. Soon afterward tiny blister-like lesions appear in the area. After about
48 hours these lesions crust over. The infection runs its course in seven to
ten days, but in about one percent of individuals it is recurrent. The recurrence is not felt to be a reinfection, but a latent infection which becomes
active under favorable conditions. Colds, respiratory tract infections, reactions to food or drugs, sunburn, fever, physical injury, stress, and menstrual
periods are all predisposing factors.

Lesions most frequently occur on the lips, around the mouth, and
other areas of the face. The lower lip is more frequently involved than the
upper lip, and individuals with recurrent infections tend to have them in
the same location. Herpes simplex (Herpes I) may occasionally occur in
the lower trunk or genital areas, but is self-limiting and does not cause recurrent genital herpes as may be seen with the Herpes II virus.

## TREATMENT

1. Within 24 hours of the onset of the first symptoms the application of an
   ice cube to the area for 45-60 minutes will abort the fever blister. Ting-

ling, pain, and burning cease almost immediately and within 24 hours the blisterlike lesions are reabsorbed. Healing is complete within one to two days. This form of treatment is not effective if delayed more than 24 hours after onset of symptoms. (212, 213)

2. Avoid overexposure to sun and sunburn.

3. Avoid foods you may be allergic to. We have received several reports that people who eliminated chocolate from their diet had no further fever blister outbreaks.

4. Regular out-of-doors exercise will reduce stress, and will strengthen the body to resist infection.

5. Applications of 70% alcohol will assist in drying the lesions.

6. Powdered golden seal may be applied to the fever blister. Wet the end of a toothpick as an applicator. Pain relief is rapid, and application can be repeated as often as necessary.

## FIBROCYSTIC BREAST DISEASE

Fibrocystic breast disease is the most common lesion of the female breast. It is three to four times more common than breast cancer. It generally occurs between the ages of 30 and 50, and is related to the endocrine system. Fibrocystic disease generally improves during pregnancy and nursing. It is often worse just prior to the menstrual period. It is generally active only during the reproductive years, disappearing with the menopause.

Symptoms are a feeling of discomfort, soreness or tenderness in the breast. The patient may be able to feel lumps in the breast.

Studies indicate that the risk of breast cancer is tripled in women with fibrocystic breast disease. (214)

## TREATMENT

1. Dr. John P. Minton, associate professor of surgery at Ohio State University in Columbus reports that methylxanthines (caffeine, theophylline, and theobromine) may cause breast disease. He advises women to avoid the use of coffee, tea, cola drinks and chocolate, all of which contain methylxanthines. Dr. Minton followed a group of 47 women for three years and reported that 65% of the women who eliminated these substances from their diet had complete resolution of their symptoms within six months of the dietary change. (215) Some of the women who had regression of symptoms later resumed use of coffee or other methylxanthines and had recurrence of their breast lumps. (216)

2. Nicotine also stimulates growth of breast tissue, but the metabolic pathway is apparently slightly different from that of the methylxanthines. (217)

3. Because overweight is considered a risk for breast cancer it is best to

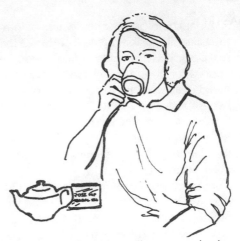

*Substitute herbal beverages and teas for coffee, tea, and colas*

keep the weight low. Tumors in a large breast are more difficult to find than in a small breast.

4. Padded bras and excess clothing of the trunk may lead to congestion of the breasts. The extremities should have as many layers of clothing as does the trunk. Overheating the breasts may increase the risk of breast disease with its increased risk of breast cancer subsequently. This may be the same way that elevating the temperature of the tests increases the risk of cancer of the testis (70 to 80 percent greater risk of cancer of the testis if it is subjected to greater heat by failure to descend from the abdomen to the scrotum).

5. Maintain adequate hydration to keep the breast secretions thin.

6. Strict regularity in breast self-examination should be practiced at least once a quarter. A good practice is to examine the breasts on each first day of a season: first day of spring, first day of summer, etc.

7. Dr. Elizabeth Bright-See, of the Ludwig Institute for Cancer Research in Toronto, reported at a seminar on nutrition and cancer in December, 1982 on a group of women with severe fibrocystic disease and strong family history of cancer. They were put on a very low fat (especially animal fat) diet; preliminary results showed marked improvement in only six months. (A control diet, high in meat, milk, eggs, butter and cheese, consumed by reluctant medical students was facetiously referred to as "the suicide diet.")

8. A recent study from Canada points out high estrogen levels found in milk and dairy products. The implications for both fibrocystic disease and potential breast cancer are not lost upon the authors. They suggest a diet free of dairy products, even eliminating them in cooking.

## GASTROENTERITIS

Gastroenteritis, also called "stomach flu," is an inflammation of the gastrointestinal tract. It may be due to bacterial or viral infection, chemical irritation, allergies, some medications, or emotional stresses.

Symptoms are fever, nausea and vomiting, diarrhea, muscle aches and abdominal pain. Acute symptoms generally do not last longer than 24-48 hours.

Most cases of gastroenteritis are of a viral nature, and no antibiotic treatment is effective; in fact, antibiotics are one of the commonest causes of serious gastroenteritis.

Onset of symptoms generally occurs within a day or two of exposure to the virus.

## TREATMENT

1. Viral gastroenteritis is contagious. Careful hygiene will assist in prevention of spread of the disease. Wash the hands frequently.
2. The treatment of choice is charcoal obtained from the pharmacy or health food store as tablets, capsules, or pulverized powder. Take eight tablets or four capsules, or one to two tablespoons of powder stirred into a glass of water. The full dosage is repeated with each vomiting episode or diarrheal stool.

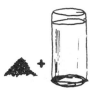

3. During the early stages of the disease, while nausea and vomiting are present, use a clear liquid diet. Ice chips may be useful in restoring lost fluids. Water is the beverage of choice, but diluted apple, grape, or cranberry juice may be used. Avoid citrus fruits and juices. Take small amounts frequently throughout the day. Do not use coffee, colas, tea, or alcoholic beverages as these all irritate the gastrointestinal tract and may induce further vomiting and/or diarrhea.
4. After vomiting and diarrhea cease, gradually begin the use of non — irritating foods such as rice, cream of wheat or cream of rice, plain cooked potatoes, apple sauce, bananas, and cooked carrots or peas. Avoid spicy foods, fatty or greasy foods, foods with a high roughage content, and milk. Whole grains, fruits with skins and/or seeds, some raw vegetables such as lettuce and celery, nuts, and foods such as corn which have hulls may all be irritating to the digestive system.
5. Bed rest may be necessary to decrease vomiting and diarrhea, and be-

cause of weakness due to fluid loss.

6. Catnip tea is very soothing to the gastrointestinal tract: one teaspoon of tea leaves to one cup of water, steeped 15 minutes, and drunk while warm. Repeat as often as needed for discomfort or nausea. Mint tea may be helpful. If it is vomited up, repeat the tea immediately after vomiting, since there is a refractory phase just after vomiting when further vomiting does not usually occur.

7. In small children and *infants*, observe closely for signs of dehydration; dry skin and mucous membranes, drowsiness, rapid respirations. If there is any question in your mind, seek medical advice!

8. In cases of inability to retain any fluids, small retention enemas of normal saline can be most helpful. Use one level teaspoon of salt per pint of water. Using a small rubber bulb syringe, inject one to two ounces of the solution into the rectum and hold the buttocks together for several minutes. Repeat every one to two hours until improved and able to retail fluids by mouth.

## GLAUCOMA

Pressure within the eyeball (intraocular pressure) which is higher than normal is called glaucoma. Approximately one million Americans have glaucoma and do not know it. It is the cause of one-tenth of all cases of blindness, and occurs in 1 to 2.5 percent of Americans 35 years of age or older. Blindness due to glaucoma is more common in blacks than in whites. It tends to run in families. Relatives of glaucoma patients are five or six times more likely to suffer glaucoma than are persons without a history of glaucoma in the family.

Fluid is constantly being produced in the eye and constantly drains out. Pressure build-up occurs if the fluid called aqueous humor is prevented from flowing out. Normal eye pressure is about 15 to 20 millimeters of mercury, but in glaucoma levels may reach 40 millimeters of mercury or more. Picture a balloon being filled with more and more water, with none of the fluid allowed to escape. The balloon wall is subjected to increasing amounts of pressure. This increased pressure in the eyeball may lead to damage of the optic nerve producing progressive loss of vision.

There are three types of glaucoma: angle closure, open-angle, and congenital. Angle closure glaucoma is often acute in nature and a medical emergency. The patient may experience episodes of decreased vision, and colored halos around artificial lights. These episodes often occur when the person is under emotional stress or in a darkened environment which produces dilation of the pupil. There may be severe pain in or around the eye due to a rapid increase in intraocular pressure. Pain is most often present in only one eye. The pupil may become enlarged, and nausea and vomiting may be present.

Open angle glaucoma is slower in onset. The patient may experience mild discomfort or a feeling of tiredness in the eye, particularly after watching television or movies in a dark room, poor vision in dim light, and no improvement in vision with changes in prescriptions. He slowly loses his side vision – so slowly that he often does not recognize the loss. There may be halos around lights and loss of vision. This type of glaucoma is the most common. Open angle glaucoma generally begins at age 40 to 46. If untreated it may lead to blindness by age 60 to 65.

Congenital glaucoma is present at birth or shortly thereafter. It is often associated with other birth defects.

## TREATMENT

1. The person with glaucoma should be under the regular care of his physician. Early diagnosis and treatment are important in preventing blindness.
2. Worry, anger, fear, and other emotional upsets should be avoided as they may increase intraocular pressure.
3. Heavy lifting, pushing, etc. should be avoided, but moderate daily out-of-doors exercise will lower intraocular pressure.
4. Any clothing which constricts the body (tight belts, collars, girdles) may raise intraocular pressure and should be avoided.
5. Reading, sewing, etc. may be done in moderation.
6. Avoid constipation as straining at the stool increases intraocular pressure.

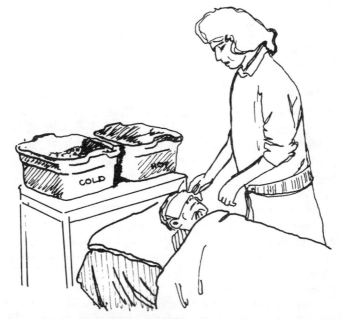

*Hot and cold compresses to the eyes may be helpful*

7. As blood pressure rises, so does intraocular pressure. Treat high blood pressure promptly and faithfully.
8. Obesity may hinder the outward flow of aqueous humor. If overweight, begin a weight reduction program.
9. A single cup of coffee is sufficient to bring on a violent glaucoma attack in susceptible persons. Avoid coffee and other caffeine-containing foods and beverages.
10. A small adhesive patch containing medication to prevent motion sickness has recently been placed on the market. Several cases of glaucoma have been induced by these patches. Other drugs such as corticosteroids (cortisone-type drugs) may induce glaucoma.
11. The new orthopedic devices that suspend a person upside-down have been shown to produce alarming elevations in both blood pressure and intraocular pressure.
12. Lying in the prone (face down) position may produce a significant increase in intraocular pressure.
13. Blood sugar abnormalities such as diabetes may hasten the onset of glaucoma.
14. Tobacco use raises intraocular pressure.
15. Do not take abnormally large amounts of fluid at one time. A glass or two at a time is probably safe. Spread fluid intake over the entire day.
16. Some believe that some cases of glaucoma may be related to a food allergy. See Appendix B for a list of the most common food allergens.
17. Hot compresses applied to the eyes for nine minutes, followed by a one minute cold compress, alternated for an hour daily may be helpful.
18. Use a sugar-free, visible-fat-free diet.

## HEMORRHOIDS

Hemorrhoids are enlarged varicose veins of the anus and rectum. Those occurring above the internal sphincter (a band of muscle fibers just inside the anus) are called internal hemorrhoids; those occurring below the internal sphincter are referred to as external hemorrhoids. External hemorrhoids are often called piles. Hemorrhoids occur most frequently between the ages of 20 and 50. (221) Symptoms may be absent for a while, then produce great discomfort.

Symptoms include bleeding, which may be severe and prolonged, even to the point of inducing anemia. Pain is sometimes so severe that the person is unable to sit or walk straight. This severe pain almost always indicates a thrombus, or clot, in one of the enlarged veins. Itching is sometimes intense but is usually mild.

Any condition which increases the intra-abdominal pressure or impairs the flow of blood through the veins of the hemorrhoidal plexus may induce hemorrhoids. Among the more common causes are constipation,

pregnancy, straining at the stool, heavy lifting, overweight, heavy coughing, frequent sneezing, prolonged use of laxatives or enemas, long periods
of either sitting or standing without moving, lack of exercise, and elevated
pressure in the portal vein of the liver as may be seen in cirrhosis of the
liver.

## TREATMENT

1. A diet high in fiber will aid in the production of soft, bulky stools which
   will pass without straining.
2. Adequate water intake is essential to avoid dry, hard stools difficult to
   pass.
3. Daily out-of-doors exercise will stimulate normal bowel function.
4. Sitz baths may bring pain relief. Sit in hot water ten to twelve inches
   deep at 100 degrees F. for 10 to 20 minutes three to five times a day.
   Spreading the buttocks apart may enable the water more ready access
   to the area. Fold a large towel to form a cushion to sit on in the tub. The
   sitz bath will soothe inflamed tissues and relax the spasms of the anal
   and rectal muscles which often accompany the inflammation.

   A quarter-cup of witch hazel may be added to the sitz bath if
desired.

   In severe cases, alternating hot and cold sitz baths can be used.
One way is to use two large galvanized wash tubs, propped up at an
angle for comfortable sitting. One should be filled with hot water, and
the other with tap water. Sit in the hot tub for five minutes and the cold
one for 30 seconds to one minute. Alternate the hot and cold three
times.

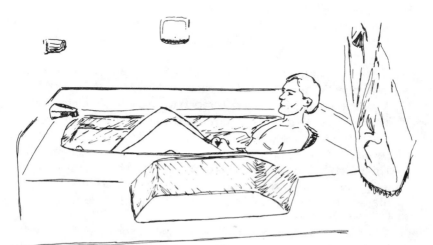

5. Avoid spicy, highly seasoned foods such as chili and pizza, as these may irritate the already inflamed area.
6. A mild laxative action may be desired but this should be very gentle. Diarrhea will greatly aggravate the problem. Oatmeal, whole wheat, prunes, fruits and vegetables are all felt to have a mild laxative action.
7. Avoid excessive cleansing of the anus after a bowel movement. Patting with slightly dampened toilet tissue is suggested instead of rubbing. A shower could also be used.
8. Boiled onions increase the ability of the blood to clot and one person has reported that the daily intake of onions controlled bleeding. (220)
9. An ice pack may bring pain relief.
10. Compounds containing local anesthetic agents are best avoided as they may irritate the area and prolong healing. Allergic reactions to local anesthetics are common. These products often have a "caine" in the brand name or in the list of ingredients.
11. A 1976 report states that there is no evidence that any of the ingredients in Preparation H alone or with other ingredients can reduce inflammation, or shrink hemorrhoids. (222) Preparation H contains an antiseptic, a "live yeast cell derivative" and shark liver oil.
12. An astringent such as golden seal tea or witch hazel may be applied as either a hot or cold compress.
13. Avoid sitting or standing still for prolonged periods.
14. If the hemorrhoids are bleeding avoid the use of aspirin as it hinders blood clotting and will prolong the bleeding.
15. An aloe suppository may be quite effective. Cut a piece of aloe about two and a half inches long, peel, and insert.
16. Several people have reported relief with cranberry poultices. Blend a handful of cranberries in the food blender, wrap about a tablespoonful in a piece of cheesecloth to lay against the area. Change after an hour, repeating as necessary.
17. Lecithin applications may be beneficial. Simply anoint the area with a small quantity as one would vaseline.
18. A garlic bulb may be peeled, scraped to cause the juice to flow, and inserted into the rectum at bedtime. It will be expelled the next day during the normal process of elimination. (223)
19. Severe, increasing pain often indicates a thrombosed hemorrhoid. This needs to be opened and the clot removed by a physician before relief can be obtained. This is not the same thing as a hemorrhoidectomy, and is a simple, rapid treatment. Sitz baths as described above bring rapid relief.

Hemorrhoidectomy may be indicated for severely prolapsed hemorrhoids or for those that cause persistent, recurrent problems. Unnecessary discomfort and disability is often experienced by those who delay surgery for an unreasonable length of time. There are several new techniques involving rubber bands, freezing, etc. which are very satisfactory and can be done on an outpatient basis. The important thing is to find a surgeon or proctologist who is very familiar and proficient with the procedure.

## HEPATITIS (VIRAL)

Hepatitis is an inflammation of the liver. It may be caused by a virus, bacterium, or a toxic substance. We will discuss mainly the kind of hepatitis caused by a virus – viral hepatitis.

There are two main types of viral hepatitis – Hepatitis A and Hepatitis B. Hepatitis A is transmitted by contaminated water, milk, or food and has an incubation period of 15 to 45 days. The person with hepatitis is most infectious just before the onset of symptoms so food workers can transmit hepatitis before becoming ill. Generally one is free of virus within seven to nine days after jaundice (yellowing of the skin and whites of the eyes) occurs. People who work with animals may catch the virus from them. Shellfish are known carriers of hepatitis, even though the waters they are harvested from have met national sanitation standards for shellfish growing. (228). Recovery from Hepatitis A generally occurs within four weeks.

Hepatitis B is found throughout the world but is most common in areas of high population density and poor hygiene. Healthy carriers and people with active hepatitis are the major sources of infection. Hepatitis B has an incubation period of from 28 to 160 days (two to six months), and recovery may require up to six months. This type of hepatitis is felt to be most commonly transmitted by blood, but in some instances breast milk, semen and respiratory secretions are all able to transmit the virus. Contaminated needles, syringes, and other instruments may spread the virus, as may intimate contact such as kissing and sexual activity. At least six cases of hepatitis B have been traced to contaminated acupuncture needles. (230) Homosexuals who practice rectal intercourse are at high risk. Dialysis patients and those requiring blood transfusions are also at high risk. Chronic active hepatitis, which can lead to cirrhosis of the liver and death, is much more likely to occur with hepatitis B.

Symptoms of hepatitis include jaundice, fatigue, lack of appetite, headache, irritability, joint stiffness, vomiting, stomach pain, diarrhea or constipation, muscle aches, and fever. Itching or skin rashes may be present. The itching is due to the accumulation of bile salts underneath the skin. The jaundice or yellowing is first observed in the eyes and mucous membranes. The urine may become dark due to excess bilirubin being excreted by the kidneys and the stool may become clay colored because of the absence of bile pigment. The liver becomes enlarged and tender.

There are 40,000 to 70,000 cases of hepatitis reported in the United States each year, but some authorities feel that there may be ten times this number of cases which are never recognized as hepatitis. Children and young adults are most likely to have hepatitis; the highest incidence occurs in adolescent girls.

Hepatitis A has been decreasing in recent years. About 25 percent of hepatitis cases are type A. The incidence of type B hepatitis is rising with increased drug abuse in young people particularly in males 15 to 34 years of age. (229) In 1979 hepatitis ranked fourth among the 30 national communicable diseases.

## TREATMENT

1. Fortunately, most cases of hepatitis are self-limiting and will heal with rest and supportive care. Bedrest has been considered important in the treatment of hepatitis in the past, but military studies reveal that even vigorous exercise begun after the acute phase is not harmful. (231) Many authorities feel that the fatigue which accompanies the disease will limit the amount of exercise the patient feels up to, and instruct their patients to exercise but to avoid becoming overly tired. Prolonged bed rest itself can lead to weakness.

2. The patient often has a poor appetite, and sometimes even the smell of food cooking will cause him nausea. Helping these patients obtain adequate nourishment is often a challenge. Be sure the patient receives a nutritious breakfast as hepatitis patients tend to lose their appetites as the day wears on. Avoid heavy, greasy foods and alcoholic beverages. An oil-free diet is recommended.

3. Constipation should be guarded against as accumulations of stool in the large bowel allow the bloodstream to absorb more waste products such as ammonia, increasing the work load of the inflamed liver.

4. The patient should be encouraged to drink plenty of water to flush the kidneys of toxic products.

5. The patient should bathe frequently and be careful to wash the hands with soap and warm water after every bowel movement. It is best for the patient to have a separate toilet, but if this is not possible wash the toilet seat after use.

6. The patient should not prepare food for others or be in the food preparation area. He should use disposable eating utensils if possible; if not his utensils should be washed separately from those of the rest of the family. Disposable eating utensils should be placed in plastic bags for disposal.

7. Linen and personal clothing should be laundered separately.

8. The hepatitis patient should be protected from toxic fumes such as from cleaning liquids.

9. Drugs during hepatitis should be kept to a minimum as these substances are toxic to the liver. There are no antibiotics available to combat hepatitis. Birth control pills containing estrogens are known to raise the serum bilirubin levels and should not be taken. Corticosteroids

given during the acute phase may lead to later relapse, and they provide no demonstrable benefit. Even aspirin is toxic to the liver. (232)

10. Hot fomentations over the liver area for 15 minutes followed by a cold
    sponging, repeating the alternating hot and cold for four repetitions
    may be done on a daily basis. Finish the treatment with a shower or
    sponge bath.

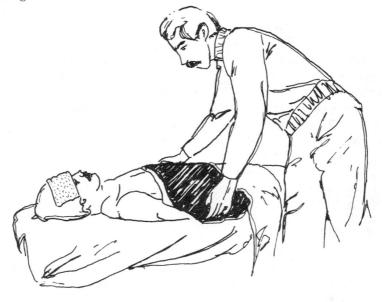

11. A hot half bath may be given to raise the body temperature and assist
    the body in fighting the virus. The patient sits in a tub of water as hot
    as can be tolerated until the body temperature reaches 102 to 104 de-
    grees F. The water temperature may then be cooled to maintain this
    temperature for approximately twenty minutes. Apply washcloths
    wrung from ice water to the face and head to keep the head cool. Give
    the patient plenty of water to drink as he will lose fluids through perspi-
    ration. After 20 minutes give a cool shower, dress the patient warmly
    and have him rest in bed until the sweating stops. The treatment may
    be given for 10 to 15 days but some patients may not be able to toler-
    ate the physical taxation of daily treatments.

## HIATUS HERNIA

Hiatus hernia refers to a protrusion of part of the stomach into the
chest cavity through the diaphragm. A weakness in the diaphragm as it fits
around the esophagus may enlarge the opening for the esophagus, leaving
room for the stomach to slide up. The weakness is often caused by increased pressure in the abdominal cavity. Obesity, pregnancy, tumors,

tight clothing, heavy lifting, coughing, overeating, and straining at the stool are all known to increase intra-abdominal pressure. Aging, lack of exercise, poor nutrition, injury, and extended periods in bed such as with a prolonged illness may also be predisposing factors.

Hiatus hernia is the most common abnormality of structure of the upper gastrointestinal tract and many people are unaware that they have a hiatus hernia. Some studies suggest that hiatus hernia can be demonstrated in over 20 percent of North American adults on x-ray studies. (225)

Heartburn is probably the most common symptom and is due to irritation of the esophagus by acids from the stomach. Difficulty swallowing and the sudden return of material from the stomach into the throat or mouth are also common. This material is often described as tasting hot, sour, or bitter. There may be a sensation of a lump in the throat or a feeling that food sticks in the throat. Over a prolonged period, this may cause chronic esophagitis, leading to marked difficulty in swallowing and strictures of the esophagus.

Hiatus hernia occurs in women four times as often as in men, perhaps due to their tight clothing. They occur most often in the 40 to 70 year old group. (224)

## TREATMENT

1. Avoid constipation by using a wide variety of whole grains, fruits, and vegetables. Avoid all refined foods including white flour products and sugar. It may be necessary to add one to three tablespoons of bran to the daily diet.
2. Drink six to eight glasses of water daily.
3. Avoid overeating.
4. A two meal a day program (breakfast and lunch) is better than three meals; if supper is eaten it should be light (fruit and whole grains) and two to three hours before bedtime. Food in the stomach when one lies down is likely to flow back up into the throat. Omission of supper may be the single best treatment for heartburn.
5. Overweight persons should reduce their weight normal to or slightly below.
6. Avoid tight clothing such as corsets, girdles, belts, and tight bands.
7. If a person has much discomfort during the night raising the head of the bed with four to eight inch blocks may be helpful.
8. The use of aloe vera juice or gel, two ounces every two hours as necessary, may provide good symptomatic relief of heartburn. Finely ground slippery elm powder, two teaspoons dissolved in a little water as needed can be very soothing.
9. Daily out-of-doors exercise will assist in producing good muscle tone and help prevent constipation. Walking and gardening are excellent. Avoid strenuous exercise after meals.

10. Avoid heavy lifting, straining, or bending immediately after meals.
11. Stress often induces symptoms and should be avoided. (224) Exercise neutralizes stress.
12. Food should be eaten on a regular schedule to allow the stomach to empty properly before the next meal. Do not eat between meals as this delays stomach emptying.
13. The lower end of the esophagus normally has an area called the esophageal sphincter, that acts as a barrier to prevent irritating stomach acid and contents from refluxing (washing up) into the esophagus. Some foods, drugs, and tobacco (either smoked or chewed) are known to decrease lower esophageal sphincter pressure, increasing acid reflux from the stomach into the esophagus, and resulting in heartburn. Offending substances include the methylxanthines (found in coffee and chocolate), alcohol, citrus juices, spicy foods, tomato, tobacco, peppermint, and spearmint. Avoid these items. Coffee is particularly bad as the decrease in lower esophageal sphincter pressure occurs during the first 30 to 45 minutes after intake of the coffee, since acid production in the stomach due to coffee's stimulating effect is at a peak at this same time, reflux and heartburn are often severe. (226) Whole milk also produces significant reductions in lower esophageal sphincter pressure. (227)
14. Tobacco is such a potent paralyzer of the lower esophageal sphincter that one puff of a cigarette may lower sphincter pressure to zero. Stomach contents can then wash freely into the esophagus, producing the well-known "smoker's heartburn." Not only will tobacco use markedly aggravate hiatus hernia, but it may be responsible for all of the symptoms of the hernia without actually having one. The only remedy is stopping the use of tobacco.

## HYPERACTIVE CHILD

Hyperactivity is a very common childhood problem today and causes major difficulties in many American homes. Almost all children display overactive behavior at one time or another during their life.

The hyperactive child squirms and fidgets, cannot remain seated for any period of time, runs instead of walks, and constantly goes from one thing to another. Many hyperactive children never stop talking. Their attention span is short, they act before thinking, are impulsive, easily distracted, and forget easily. They are often unable to follow a series of instructions and have a low frustration level. They are often moody, irritated, easily upset, and have difficulty concentrating.

A portion of cases of hyperactivity are due to emotional problems or to intelligence levels. A portion are due to inadequate, inconsistent, or ineffective discipline in the home. Hyperactive children often control the situation in their homes more than do the parents; parents often yield to the child's wishes to avoid a confrontation. Children who are often disciplined by screaming parents soon stop listening and become uncontrollable. Parents must control their own behaviors in order to have control of their children.

Spoiled children have greater control of home situations than do their parents. When this child enters school where there are controls placed on his behavior, he often manifests overactive behavior in an attempt to control this environment as well. Parents must remember that children require discipline.

A developmental deviation or lag accounts for one type of hyperactivity. These children are unable to control their behavior, as their "control center" does not develop as rapidly as does the motor division of the body. Controls catch up with motor activity by puberty, and the level of activity decreases; concentration and attention span improve.

Learning disabilities are often observed in hyperactive children. These learning disabilities are also due to developmental lags and may be outgrown with time. This type of child may be able to repair his own bike or assemble complicated models, but unable to learn to read. Many educators are now suggesting that children not be sent to school until they are eight to ten years of age, to allow time for fine muscle coordination to develop. Boys suffer from learning disabilities more frequently than girls, because until puberty their development is slower than that of girls.

Overstimulation from television, competitive games, etc. may lead to hyperactivity. Some psychiatrists feel that the constant change of visual frames seen in television shows, as well as the content of violence in many programs has a stimulating effect on sensitive children. With the frequent change of scenes the view is trained to a short attention span. Children with overtaxed nervous systems often indulge in unfocused activity and irritability. This probably explains why a guided exercise program directed toward the large muscles of the body was shown effective in calming hyperactive children. We feel that gardening, yard work, and similar activities carried out with the parents will be very beneficial to the hyperactive child.

A child is three times more likely to be hyperactive if his mother smokes 23 or more cigarettes a day during the pregnancy than if she does not smoke at all. The reasons for this are not clearly understood, but it may be that the decrease in blood flow to the placenta which occurs in smokers may retard the development of the fetus.

Dr. John Ott believes that certain types of fluorescent lights are stimulating, and he cites studies in which a group of students in a classroom demonstrated behavior improvement when the type of lighting in their classroom was changed. However, this theory needs further study before it can be definitely cited as a cause of hyperactivity.

Some hyperactive children are easily identified, even as infants. They may have difficulty sleeping or eating (they often have colic), and they frequently crawl out of the their cribs. When they begin crawling these children seem to keep their parents constantly on the run trying to keep them out of things. They may get up during the night and get into things. They may show reactions to medication the opposite of what one would expect; medications given to calm other children may keep these children up all night. They manifest peer problems as they mature. They may play well with one child, but with more than one playmate arguments often break out. They usually try to control their playmates. This is cited as another reason to delay the school enrollment and instruct these children at home, especially boys.

That a major effort to correct hyperactivity and out-of-control children should be made early in life is evidenced by the fact that a high percentage of these children grow up to be troubled teenagers with serious problems – drugs, dropouts, depressions, crimes, etc.

Undoubtedly the majority of cases of hyperactivity are due to nutritional factors as discussed later.

## TREATMENT

1. Regardless of the reasons for their hyperactivity, overactive children respond favorably to a structured and predictable environment. The more consistency in the environment, the greater the decrease in overactivity.

2. Consistency is the key in the management of hyperactive children. For child management to be effective the child must know that the parent means what he says. Threats like "If you do that one more time I will break both your arms," obviously will not be carried out, and the child, knowing that the parent will not actually do as he says, finds it easy to believe that he will not carry out other disciplinary measures. Overstatements train the child to disobedience, because he knows that the parent doesn't mean what he says.

   Changing one's mind after giving instructions to a child leads to a fluid, unstable environment. A mother telling her child to go take his bath may be met with such resistance from the child that she decides to let him go to bed without his bath. The child learns that he can force the parent to change his or her mind.

   The parent of an overactive child must check to be certain that his child has actually done what he was instructed to do. If the child knows the parents will not check he may not follow instructions, but may tell his parents that he has.

   The best book in print on the subject of child management is a book called CHILD GUIDANCE by E. G. White; Review and Herald Publishers, Washington, D.C.

3. Another reason to check whether or not the child has carried out instructions is that this type of child is easily distracted and forgets what

he was supposed to do. The child must be trained to remember.
4. Parents must present a united front to their child. They must have set rules and expectations. When one parent undermines the other, confusion and unpredictability result, which may be expected to increase overactivity in the child. Additionally, the child is able to play one parent against the other to get his own way.

There is a strong impression, though definite studies may be lacking, that children from broken homes are more likely to have behavioral problems such as hyperactivity.
5. A regular schedule is vital in the management of hyperactive children. Rising time, meals, and bedtime should be at a set time 365 days a year. A child who is accustomed to going to bed at a set time will resist less than a child who has an irregular bedtime. Established routines make the environment more stable.
6. When setting rules for children, parents should also state the punishment if the rule is broken. This enables the child to know what the consequences of misbehavior will be. If the child knows that the parent will enforce the rule he comes to understand that he is responsible for his own behavior, and that the things that result from it – good or bad – are caused by him.
7. Some children misbehave to gain attention. In many homes the only time a child's behavior is noticed is when he is misbehaving. Parents often pay more attention to mistakes, shortcomings, and failures than to successes and achievements. Not reacting to misbehavior is an effective method of discipline if properly used. Behavior that disturbs others or may produce damage to people or property cannot be safely ignored, but temper tantrums, pouting, whining, etc. are often best ignored. Often when the child observes that the parent is ignoring his behavior he will intensify it, but this increase should last not more than five days at the most. As the child sees that the parent does not react even to this increase in inappropriate behavior, he will give it up.

Recognizing a child's good behavior tends to reinforce it. If the child cleans his room, runs an errand without complaining, etc. he should be commended for it.

## DIET

8. The Feingold diet has been useful in many cases of hyperactivity. This diet eliminates all foods containing salicylates.

### SALICYLATE-CONTAINING FOODS

| | |
|---|---|
| Almonds | Cherries |
| Apples | Cucumbers |
| Apricots | Currants |
| Blackberries | Gooseberries |
| Boysenberries | Grapes |

Nectarines Oranges Peaches Pickles Plums Prunes Raisins Raspberries Strawberries Tomatoes

Foods containing BHT, artificial colors, and flavors must also be eliminated. If, after four to six weeks, the child shows a favorable response to the diet, foods in the above list may be reintroduced to the diet, one at a time. If no increase in activity is noted after three or four days of using the food, another food may be added. Test all foods in this fashion.

The diet must be strictly followed. Even a slight breakover may nullify the benefits of the diet.

Dr. Feingold suggests that the whole family go on the diet at the same time. This makes it easier for mother and child. For a good discussion on this subject see the book FOOD ALLERGIES MADE SIMPLE by Austin, Thrash and Thrash.

Food allergy is felt by many researchers to be a frequent cause of hyperactivity. Sugar and milk are considered the chief offenders, but eggs, corn, wheat, citrus, beef and pork are all frequent causes of allergic reactions. Foods that irritate the stomach or inflame the nerves must be removed from the child's dietary. That would include coffee, tea, colas, and chocolate; any vinegar products, cheese, sauerkraut, soy sauce, miso and any fermented food; baking soda and baking powder products; and most foods having very strong or pungent flavors such as spices. Sweets and highly refined carbohydrates should be strictly prohibited. They can be replaced by natural foods such as the whole grain products, both breads and cereals; vegetables and fresh fruits (fruits canned without sugar are usually acceptable); with beans and other legumes. These foods provide an abundance of the nerve-calming B-vitamins and minerals, whereas highly refined "junk foods" not only tend to be deficient in these essential nutrients but also require more of them to be metabolized. It can readily be appreciated that the diet must involve a thorough reformation of the kitchen and management of spending money. A superficial attempt to reform is doomed to failure and has led many to believe diet is uninvolved in hyperactivity, whereas in truth it is a principal factor.

## MEDICATIONS

9. Medications commonly given for hyperactivity may produce loss of appetite, muscle stiffness, shaking, trembling, dizziness, constipation, insomnia, headaches, stomach aches, and increased nervous behaviors such as nail biting. Some children develop allergies. There are studies suggesting that these medications also produce growth suppression. Many feel that medications should be used for hyperactivity only as a last resort. It takes from the child the responsibility for his own behavior, and serves as a crutch.

## HYPERTENSION (HIGH BLOOD PRESSURE)

Hypertension, commonly called high blood pressure, is a sustained increase in the pressure in the blood vessels. Blood pressure is generally recorded in two figures. The first is the systolic pressure, the pressure built up when the heart muscle pumps blood out of the heart into the aorta. The pressure is measured by the distance in millimeters that it will raise a column of mercury. Between beats, as the heart relaxes, the pressure drops. The pressure immediately before the heart contracts again is called the diastolic pressure.

Systolic hypertension appears to be due to loss of elastic tissue and to arteriosclerotic changes in the large blood vessels. These changes are often the result of the aging process, as well as to dietary, hereditary, and lifestyle factors. Emotional stress also influences the systolic pressure. Enlargement of the heart, coronary artery disease, and strokes are associated with an elevated systolic blood pressure.

Diastolic hypertension results from a decrease in the size of the arterioles (tiny blood vessels) and increased blood viscosity (thickness).

Hypertension may produce no symptoms and its presence be unsuspected. Other persons experience headache, blurred vision, difficulty breathing or a feeling of giddiness.

Primary, or essential, hypertension is hypertension whose cause is not understood. Approximately 90 percent of all hypertension falls in this category. Secondary hypertension occurs as a result of other diseases.

Primary hypertension is felt to occur in one out of ten persons living in the United States today. Approximately 60,000 persons die each year as the result of longstanding high blood pressure which induces hypertensive heart disease.

Hypertension is the primary risk factor for stroke and one of three risk factors for myocardial infarctions (heart attacks) and coronary artery disease (disease of the blood vessels of the heart).

When compared to people with normal blood pressure, patients with blood pressure higher than 160 systolic and 95 diastolic had a three-fold risk for coronary disease and peripheral vascular disease, a four-fold risk for congestive heart failure and a seven-fold risk of stroke! (234)

It is estimated that half of the population suffering from high blood pressure are not even aware that they have it, and of those who have been diagnosed, only a few are being adequately treated.

Primary hypertension most often occurs in middle aged and older persons, although it is found in young people and even infants. Women develop hypertension more frequently than do men, but men are more dramatically affected by longstanding elevation of the blood pressure. In the United States blacks develop hypertension more readily than do whites. People living in stressful urban areas develop high blood pressure more frequently than those living in rural areas. Overweight individuals are particularly susceptible and a reduction in weight is often adequate to control blood pressure.

**TREATMENT**

1. For many years lowering sodium (salt) intake has been known to be effective in controlling hypertension. Some people are much more sensitive to salt than are others, but most Americans consume far too much salt. Most convenience and snack foods are high in salt. The following are some simple guidelines used by Dr. Lewis Dahl to reduce daily salt intake to less than 1000 mg.:
   A.  Never add salt to the food in cooking.
   B.  Do not add salt at the table.
   C.  Eliminate all dairy products as they are all high in sodium.
   D.  All processed meats are high in salt and should be eliminated.
   E.  Use no canned vegetables unless home canned without salt as commercially canned vegetables all contain salt. Watch for other sources of sodium such as monosodium glutamate in food, drugs, vending machine food and drink, frozen food, and all other sources.
2. Many studies have shown a correlation between body weight and blood pressure, and the correlation is strongest in young and middle-aged persons. Loss of weight lowers blood pressure. Dr. Hans Selye, the world authority on stress states that overeating aggravates hypertension in most cases. A group of overweight hypertensives were given no medication but placed on a weight reduction program. They were allowed a normal salt intake. Seventy-five percent of the group returned to normal blood pressure. (233)
3. Such factors as stress, anger, fear, and pain increase blood pressure. Control stress with adequate daily out-of-doors exercise. Exercise will also assist in clearing fats from the blood. Running in place for six minutes daily helps reduce blood pressure.
4. A low fat diet will decrease blood viscosity, lowering blood pressure. Eliminate all free fats including fried foods, cooking and salad oils, mayonnaise and margarine. (Any fat added to food is called a free fat.)
5. Studies at the Louisiana State Medical School reveal that sugar raises blood pressure. Monkeys given salt and sugar in amounts typically eaten by many Americans demonstrated higher blood pressure than monkeys given only salt. (235)
6. Persons who normally consume a high fiber diet have shown lower blood pressures. A group of patients who normally ate a low fiber diet, given a high fiber diet for a month, demonstrated lower blood pressure levels. (236)
7. Vegetarians were reported in 1974 to have lower blood pressure than

meat eaters. (237) Differences in blood pressures between vegetarians and meat eaters increase with advancing age. (238) Pork has been known for years to induce hypertension. (239)

8. Garlic lowers blood pressure probably by dilating blood vessels. (240)
9. Dietary potassium has been shown to have an anti-hypertensive effect. (241) Cereals, fruits, and vegetables are high in potassium.
10. That proper dress is important in the treatment of hypertension, is demonstrated by the "cold pressor test." The blood pressure is taken, then the subject immerses his hand in ice water for five to ten minutes. The blood pressure in very sensitive persons may rise from 40 to 100 points. A group of subjects waiting undressed in cold air showed significant increases in systolic blood pressures. (242) Dress at all times to keep the extremities as warm as the trunk.
11. Sunbathing lowers blood pressure. (243) The maximal effect occurs in about 24 hours and lasts for several days. Be careful to avoid sunburn.
12. Coffee, cigarettes, and alcohol all increase blood pressure and should be eliminated. (244, 245, 246)
13. Both systolic and diastolic blood pressures are lower in people who regularly attend religious services. (247)
14. All blood pressure medications have adverse effects, but the proper diet, exercise, and rest will in most cases make the medication unnecessary.

## INFECTIOUS MONONUCLEOSIS

Infectious momonucleosis is an acute infection caused by the Epstein-Barr virus. The infection, also called "kissing disease," is common in children, adolescents, and young adults. Infectious mononucleosis occurs early in life in underdeveloped countries, but it is usually undiagnosed: when it occurs in older children and young adulthood it is more likely to be diagnosed. Infectious mononucleosis is a self-limiting disease.

In the United States college students seem to have the disease in greatest numbers in the early fall and spring. It is estimated that about 12 percent of susceptible college students will become infected. The disease is spread by saliva, intimate personal contact and blood transfusions. Adults are believed to have an incubation period of 30 to 50 days, but in young children the incubation period may range from 4 to 14 days.

For four to five days prior to the onset of full-blown symptoms the patient may suffer from fatigue and headache. The symptoms progress to fever of 100 to 103 degrees F. (257), sore throat, and enlarged lymph glands, especially in the neck. The pharynx and tonsils are often covered with a thick, tenacious white exudate, or "membrane;" strep throat or diphtheria may be confused with it at this stage. The patient may be almost unable to swallow. In adults the fever may persist for seven to ten days. Children experience little or no fever with this disease. Approximately half of infectious mononucleosis patients have palpable enlargement of the spleen. There may be swelling of the eyelids, muscle aches, nausea, vomiting, light sensitivity and skin rash. Serious complications occur, but fortunately are rare.

## TREATMENT

1. Rest and patience are the best therapy for infectious mononucleosis. The acute phase generally lasts about two weeks but complete recovery may take several months. The patient should spend most of his time resting until the fever subsides. Activity resumption should be gradual; the patient should be as active as he feels capable of without undue fatigue.

    The patient should not indulge in heavy lifting, competitive sports and strenuous exercise as exertion or trauma may cause rupture of the spleen. (258)
2. Luella Doub, who practiced hydrotherapy for many years, states that 30 minutes of fever therapy daily for three days, maintaining the body temperature at 102 to 103 degrees F., was adequate to treat even the most advanced cases of infectious mononucleosis. (259) In our experience, the hot bath fever therapy has produced almost as dramatic results as the use of corticosteroids, with none of their drawbacks.
3. Corticosteroids have been given in the past, but these medications impair immunologic function (260) and should not be used. They do not alter the course of the disease. Antimicrobial agents (antibiotics) also fail to influence the course of the disease, (261) but do introduce another potentially injurious factor.
4. It is not necessary to isolate the patient but intimate contact, common use of drinking straws, glasses, and cups should be prohibited.
5. Warm or hot salt water gargles or irrigations may be used every hour if needed for sore throat.
6. Drink plenty of fluids to assist the kidneys in eliminating toxins.
7. The diet should be light, and free from sugar and fats.

## INSOMNIA

Almost 100 million Americans occasionally suffer from insomnia and another 20 million complain of chronic sleep problems. Seven or eight times more women than men report sleep difficulties. Americans take about 600 tons of sleeping pills a year. Sleeping pill sales are second only to aspirin in this country. Side effects from sleeping medications include depression, skin rashs, anxiety, irritability, poor coordination, loss of appetite, digestive disturbances, disorders of blood circulation and respiration, breakdown of some parts of the blood such as white blood cells which help the body resist infections, difficulty with vision, high blood pressure, liver and kidney problems, damage to the central nervous system, memory loss, dizziness and confusion. They may also lead to insomnia!

Sleep requirements vary from person to person. Many people who worry over being unable to sleep are merely trying to force the body to sleep more than it requires. Some people require only six hours of sleep per night, others need ten. If you can sleep six hours a night and not feel fatigue the next day, you are an efficient sleeper and have more waking hours for productive activities.

Sleep requirements may temporarily change. During illness, pregnancy, or stress a person may need more sleep; with a sense of well-being less sleep may be required. Interestingly, during periods of weight gain more sleep appears to be needed; during weight loss less seems required.

Personality and sleep requirements are apparently related. Short sleepers seem to be outgoing, lively, more contented and more efficient; while long sleepers tend to worry about things, be introverted, depressed and anxious.

Many people who complain of insomnia and report little or no sleep may actually sleep much more than they think. Apparently some people dream about not sleeping and awaken feeling that they really have not slept. Others, who drift between stages 0, 1 and 2 of sleep, sleep lightly but feel that they did not sleep at all.

There are four stages of sleep which we will discuss later, and two types of sleep – REM and NREM. REM (rapid-eye-movement) sleep is characterized by paralysis of the large muscles, twitching of facial muscles, fingers and toes, and generally cessation of snoring. The heart rate is faster than during NREM sleep, blood pressure and pulse higher, and brain temperature increased. There may be irregular breathing. About 80 percent of the time spent in REM sleep is felt to be spent dreaming.

During NREM (non-rapid-eye-movement) sleep the body's metabolism slows. Most of the restorative activities of the body occur during NREM sleep. Growth hormone levels in the blood stream increase during this type of sleep.

## SLEEP STAGES

Stage 0 is a state of relaxed wakefulness. The electroencephalogram (EEG, a machine which traces brain waves) shows a rhythm of ten cycles per second, but should the person open his eyes or put forth mental effort to solve a problem the rhythm changes. When the person falls asleep he enters Stage I which is NREM sleep, and EEG waves become fast, very small and irregular. This is a light sleep and the person is easily awakened during this stage.

The sleeper descends into Stage 2 NREM sleep. The senses are diminished during this phase, heart and respiratory rates slow, temperature drops, and oxygen consumption decreases.

Twenty to forty minutes after onset of sleep Stage 3 begins. In this stage it is difficult to awaken the sleeper and body processes continue to to slow. Stage 4 begins about ten minutes after Stage 3. The EEG during Stages 3 and 4 shows what are called delta waves – large, slow waves of one to two cycles per second. Stage 4 is the deepest sleep, and anyone awakened during this stage will be temporarily confused.

Within an hour of falling asleep the sleeper rapidly progresses back through Stages 3 and 2, to enter REM or dream sleep. The first REM sleep lasts only five to ten minutes. The first sleep cycle (Stages 1, 2, 3, 4, 3, 2 and REM) are completed 70 to 80 minutes after falling asleep. This cycle is repeated four to five times a night. The second cycle usually lasts about 110 minutes and the third cycle about 120 minutes, but the later cycles are shorter, approximately 90 minutes each. The average adult is in Stage 2 sleep for about half of the night. Delta and REM sleep make up most of the balance of the sleep time.

## TREATMENT

1. Regularity is probably the key to good sleep. Without a regular bedtime and rising time the body loses its normal rhythmic fall and rise in body temperature which contributes to wakefulness or sleepiness. One study revealed that people with regular habits had faster reaction times and were happier than people with irregular sleeping times. Irregular hours may even cause you to feel tired and unrefreshed after a night's sleep. Arising at the same time every morning will assist in falling asleep at the same time every night. Sleeping in on week-ends and holidays disrupts the biological clock, leading to increased sleeping problems.

2. Daytime naps disrupt the biological clock by making it more difficult to fall asleep at night. Going to bed early should be avoided as the person will probably be unable to sleep and will toss and turn, becoming more and more concerned over their inability to fall asleep.

3. If unable to sleep after going to bed, get up and read or carry on quiet, relaxing activities until you are sleepy. You may feel sleepy the next day, but do not nap.

4. Do not use over-the-counter sleep aids. Most of them are made up of antihistamines, pain relievers, bromides and/or scopolamine. They are often ineffective and have unwanted side-effects.

5. Alcohol, barbiturates and most hypnotics used to induce sleep suppress REM sleep. The continual use of sleeping medications often worsens sleep problems rather than solving them because people are often drowsy during the day. The person may take a daytime nap which makes nighttime sleep slower in coming.

6. Room temperature probably should be between 60 and 65 degrees. Dreams seem to be more unpleasant in rooms that are too cold, but in a room too warm people move about more and awaken more frequently.

7. The noise of a fan or air conditioner may mask noises that would otherwise disturb sleep.
8. Exercise is essential to the best sleep. Athletes have more delta sleep
   than those who do not exercise. Skipping exercise for the day affects
   that night's sleep. Exercise should not be done just prior to bedtime as
   it stimulates the body and will slow the onset of sleep.
9. Caffeine and tobacco both interfere with sleep. A one-pack-a-day
   smoker stays awake about 19 minutes more per night than the nonsmoker. Smokers who smoke three packs a day fall asleep more slowly,
   wake more often, and have less stage 4 and REM sleep than non-
   smokers. Sleep patterns begin to improve within three days of stopping the use of tobacco and after two weeks stage 4 and REM sleep
   patterns are normal.
10. Monosodium glutamate (MSG) may induce insomnia.
11. The hypoglycemic syndrome may lead to sleep problems. We recom-
    mend the health recovery program (See Appendix A).
12. Overeating interferes with sleep, particularly in the evening. Be mod-
    erate in all things. Excessive demands are made on the body anytime
    one overeats. Food should be eaten slowly and chewed thoroughly.
    The digestive system should be allowed to rest along with the rest of
    the body.
13. Many people are stimulated by fatty foods, sugar, white flour, salt,
    chemical preservatives, additives, and any food they are allergic to. See
    Appendix B for a list of the most common food allergens. Use as many
    fresh foods as possible, avoiding processed foods.
14. L-tryptophan has been widely promoted as an aid to sleep. Recent
    studies show that tryptophan taken in a concentrated form can have
    very different effects on the body than when taken in its natural form.
    There are suggestions that toxicity may result from either short or long
    term use of tryptophan in a concentrated form.
15. Herbal teas such as catnip, hops and chamomile may be used occa-
    sionally for sleep problems.
16. Check your mattress for comfort. It may be time to invest in a new mat-
    tress and a new outlook on sleep. A mattress should have a coil count
    of at least 300 coils for every 54 inches of mattress. Look for a mattress
    with a long warranty as this usually suggests a better built product.
17. Ensure an adequate supply of fresh air in the bedroom during sleeping
    hours, but avoid drafts. You breathe in over 25 barrels of air per night
    and you should see that it is the best available.
18. Everything you have done, said, felt, thought, eaten or drunk during
    the day affects what happens when you lie down at night to sleep.
    Keep the thoughts focused heavenward during the day and eat and
    drink to the glory of your loving Father.

## LICE

There are three types of lice which infect man – Pediculosis capitis (head louse), P. corporis (body louse) and P. pubis (crab louse).

Head lice are usually found on the scalp and hair at the back of the head and behind the ears. Children and people with long hair are most frequently infested. The tiny nits (eggs) are laid at the base of a hair shaft; as the hair grows the firmly attached egg moves away from the scalp. Itching and the appearance of lice and eggs are the most common symptoms.

Head lice may be spread by coats hung together, caps, scarves, carpets, upholstered furniture, bedding, combs, brushes, etc.

Adult lice live about 30 days. The female may lay about ten eggs per day, producing hundreds of offspring.

Body lice live mainly in the clothing, chiefly in the seams. They migrate onto the body for their twice a day feedings.

Crab lice are transmitted chiefly by sexual contact and are generally localized to the genital region. The chief symptom is itching. Inspection reveals tiny black or rust-colored dots clinging to the base of the hairs. The lice may spread to infest the hairs of the chest, beard, and eyelashes.

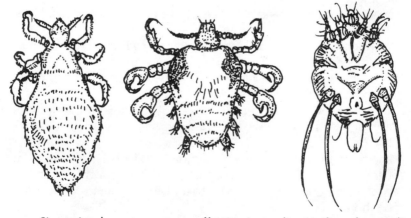

Since simple measures are effective in eradicating lice, there is little justification for using toxic pharmacologic agents. Lindane (Kwell) and pyrethrins (RID) are the two most widely used treatments for lice. Lindane has been reported to induce convulsions. The Environmental Protection Agency has suggested that lindane (Kwell) be banned as it is reported to cause cancer, birth defects, nerve damage and aplastic anemia. (262) Pyrethrins (RID) are also toxic, irritating to the mucous membranes and eyes. Allergic reactions have been reported. It is especially harmful to those sensitive to ragweed pollen.

## TREATMENT

1. Body lice may be eradicated by laundering the clothing and bedding

in hot water. A 30 minute very warm soaking bath with soap will kill any lice which may be on the body. The lice are generally on the body only for feedings, then return to the clothing. Body lice will leave a person with a fever, or one overheated by exercise.

2. Sprays are sometimes recommended for use on carpets, furniture, etc. but they are no more effective than vacuuming.

3. Combs and brushes may be soaked for an hour in 2 percent Lysol, heated in water to a temperature of about 66 C. (151 F.) for five to ten minutes, or frozen for about 30 minutes.

4. Bedding and clothing should be washed and dried in the hot cycle of the washer and dryer. Unwashable items may be deloused by sealing in a plastic bag for ten days.

5. Dousing the hair with kerosene and wrapping it in a towel is an old remedy.

6. Toilet seats should be scrubbed frequently and carpets and upholstered furniture vacuumed frequently.

7. Flowers of sulfur compresses may be used.

8. Garlic compresses applied directly to the scalp and worn for two hours are smelly but effective.

9. Equal parts of olive oil and kerosene may be applied to the scalp to get rid of the eggs.

10. Hot vinegar applied to the scalp may loosen eggs and allow them to be combed from the hair with a fine-toothed comb.

11. A 1:1 vinegar-water rinse followed by vigorous combing with a fine-toothed comb will assist in nit removal. (263)

12. Lice of eyebrows may be treated with petrolatum applied thickly twice daily for eight days, followed by combing with a fine-toothed comb. (264)

13. Pennyroyal oil mixed with an equal amount of alcohol may be dabbed on the scalp of the patient. Rub it into the scalp thoroughly, especially about the hairline and ears; allow it to remain ten minutes, then shampoo thoroughly.

14. Eight grams of rue (Ruta graveolens) may be boiled in 200 gm. of water, and used to treat lice. (265)

## LUPUS

Systemic lupus erythematosus is a chronic inflammatory disease which may involve the skin, blood vessels, serous membranes (linings of the body cavities), joints, muscles, central nervous system and kidneys. The most common symptom is a butterfly-shaped rash over the nose and cheeks. This rash is reported to worsen with exposure to sun. Lupus typically runs a course of improvement between periods of worsening. It is a very complex disease and difficult to deal with. There is no known medical or surgical cure, so treatment is logically directed toward the application of simple remedies minimizing the symptoms and the hope of removing the cause or causes.

Systemic lupus erythematosus affects about one person in 400; is five to ten times more common in women than in men, and is more common in blacks than in whites. Average age of onset is about 30 years. (266)

The cause or causes of systemic lupus erythematosus are unknown. Infections, a number of drugs (including penicillin), stress, and surgery may cause a worsening of symptoms. Other common symptoms include joint pain and arthritis, fatigue, fever, weight loss, lymph gland enlargement, and a wide range of other abnormalities involving the skin, kidneys, respiratory, gastrointestinal, circulatory and central nervous systems. (268)

## TREATMENT

1. For years systemic lupus erythematosus patients have been instructed to avoid sunlight; but James Fries, in his book, "SYSTEMIC LUPUS ERYTHEMATOSUS: A CLINICAL ANALYSIS" (267) reports that this is generally unnecessary. He has observed sensitivity to sunlight in only a minority of systemic lupus erythematosus patients, and even these patients may not have this sensitivity through the entire course of their disease. He recommends graduated exposure to the sun, starting with just a few minutes, perhaps ten minutes under a shade tree on the first day out. He reports that some of his systemic lupus erythematosus patients in California are lifeguards!

   Patients who are sun-sensitive or who must be out-of-doors for longer periods than their tolerance limits should wear broad-brimmed hats, long sleeved shirts and pants. The sun's rays are less intense before 9:00 A.M. or after 4:00 P.M.

   Fluorescent lighting is a source of ultraviolet rays which may be troublesome to sensitive systemic lupus erythematosus patients. They should minimize their exposure to this light source.

2. Exercise is essential. Lack of exercise induces poor muscle tone, osteoporosis, blood clots in the lungs, muscle shrinking, and self-pity. Walking is an excellent form of exercise for this type of patient. (267) Physical therapy may be required for muscle weakness and deformities.

   Periods of depression and fatigue are common in this disease and a regular exercise program will be helpful for both of these symptoms.

3. Avoid the use of drugs. Many of them actually induce lupus-like symptoms and can be considered one of the causes of systemic lupus erythematosus. Certain types of contraceptive pills are particular offenders. Penicillin and sulfa are sensitizing drugs. Cimetidine (the most popular peptic ulcer drug) may worsen skin disease in these patients. Corticosteroids are frequently given for symptoms, but there are many troublesome side-effects, and no clearly demonstrated improvement

in the lifespan of systemic lupus erythematosus patients. The first few days there may be agitation, difficulty sleeping, and emotional changes. After a time on these medications the patient may suffer muscle wasting, central body fat accumulation, lack of ability to resist infection, bleeding in the gastrointestinal tract, osteoporosis, and mental symptoms to mention only a few. (267)

4. Hair coloring agents, hair sprays, and certain cosmetics may make the skin more sensitive to the sun and should be avoided. Wear make-up only when absolutely necessary and keep the skin clean and moist. Hair loss is common. Patients should be advised to use gentle shampoos such as baby shampoo without perfume. Permanent wave lotions should also be avoided.

5. Because lupus is so much more common in women and tends to re-

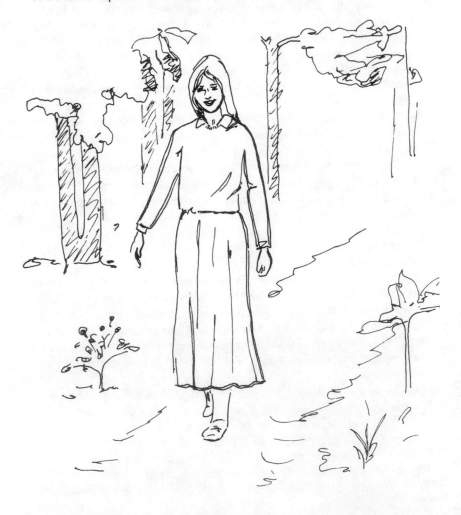

lapse after childbirth there may be an endocrine factor involved. Estrogens are found in abnormally high levels in systemic lupus erythematosus patients. For this reason we recommend a diet free from all animal foods (especially dairy products) as they may increase estrogen levels in the human body.

6. Many people with arthritis symptoms (often very prominent in lupus) are sensitive to foods in the nightshade family (potatoes, tomatoes, peppers, eggplant and tobacco). We recommend the strict elimination of these foods and their byproducts from the diet.

7. A diet free from concentrated sugars (honey, table sugar, molasses, syrups, etc.) and refined fats (fried foods, cooking fats, margarine, mayonnaise, salad dressing, etc) may be helpful.

8. It would be worth a trial of using a diet high in the natural plant sterols, ergosterol, phytosterol, sitosterol, etc. A list of such foods is given in Appendix C. Merely emphasize these foods in the diet.

9. Charcoal tablets, eight tablets midmorning, midafternoon, and at bedtime, will help remove toxins from the body. Half the dose of activated charcoal capsules will suffice, or one heaping teaspoon of the activated powder stirred into water three times a day. Charcoal constipates some people when inadequate water is drunk, and measures should be taken to relieve the condition should it occur.

10. Fever treatments to raise the body temperature to 102-103 degrees F. may be given up to five times a week if tolerated by the patient. Try to keep the temperature elevated for 20 to 30 minutes, being careful to keep the head cool by the application of ice packs or cloths wrung from ice water.

11. In some patients, heat treatments are poorly tolerated, and many of them will benefit from a short cold bath. Take a warm shower. Fill the bathtub with water from 60 to 90 degrees; and soak for three minutes. Start with the warmer temperature, and gradually decrease subsequent baths as tolerated. Always have the room warm. Physiological effects will be very similar to heat treatments.

12. A natural healing institute in Guatemala has had good success with full-body warm clay baths. We used this method on a patient with extensive skin and joint involvement with excellent results. An old bathtub filled with a thick clay paste at about 102 degrees was used outside, the patient remaining in the tub for three or four hours. We have not found an easy way to use clay inside a building.

## MEASLES (RUBEOLA)

Measles is a highly contagious disease with symptoms of fever, cough, rash, nasal discharge, itching, and inflammation of the eyes. It occurs in epidemics, most frequently during the spring. The virus is spread by droplet spray from the mouth, throat, and nose of a person coming down with the disease.

Approximately 98 percent of the population has had measles at some time during life. Infants of mothers who have had the measles appear to have an immunity for about the first year of life. (270)

The patient can infect others for two to four days before the rash appears, and remains infective for two to five days after its appearance.

The incubation period is 7 to 14 days, and the disease begins with fever, nasal discharge, cough and eye inflammation. There is commonly light sensitivity, and the face, particularly the eyes, may swell. The rash begins behind the ears, on the forehead, face and neck, and then spreads over the trunk, arms and legs. Even before the rash appears on the skin, tiny rounded, whitish spots called Koplik's spots will be seen inside the mouth. These spots help distinguish measles from other diseases, but must be searched for with the onset of fever, as they fade quickly with the appearance of the rash.

Complications of measles are dreaded, but fortunately are not usually severe in the more developed nations. They are mostly the result of secondary infection by bacteria, and consist almost exclusively of otitis media (infection of the middle ear) and pneumonia. These complications can usually be handled by very vigorous application of simple remedies, and are nearly always prevented by the treatment methods described subsequently.

**TREATMENT**

1. Antimicrobial drugs (antibiotics) should be strictly avoided, as they do not influence the course of the measles or decrease the rate of complications from measles, but do add another injurious agent for the body to fight.
2. Fluids should be encouraged, particularly during fever. The mouth may be rather sore and bland drinks and food may be soothing.
3. There is no proof that light is injurious to vision but the patient may be light sensitive and more comfortable in a darkened room.
4. Cool moisture from a vaporizer may greatly reduce cough when present.
5. Itching may be treated with Vaseline rubbed into the skin (269), aloe gel, starch or oatmeal baths. See treatment number 21 under Psoriasis for procedure.
6. Water given copiously is the best cough medicine.
7. Saline compresses applied to the eyes may be soothing. Use one teaspoon of salt to a pint of water to make normal saline solution.
8. A hot bath treatment may help relieve the fever. Place the child in a tub of hot water (105 to 108 degrees F.) about one minute for each year of his age. Be careful to keep the head cool. The treatment may be repeated every two hours. After the treatment dress the patient warmly to prevent chilling.

9. Hot fomentations to the chest may be helpful for the bronchitis which usually accompanies measles. Fomentations may be used twice a day, accompanied by a hot foot bath. A heating compress may be applied overnight.
10. Hot foot baths may be used for headache.

## MUMPS

Mumps is an infection of the salivary glands found in front of and below each ear. It rarely occurs before three years of age or after forty. Spread is by direct contact, droplets, or by contaminated articles. The typical incubation period is 16 to 18 days. The patient is infectious from two days before the swelling appears until after it disappears. Fever, pain, headache, lack of appetite, and pain in or around the ear and muscle aches may be present for one or two days before the swelling occurs. The earache may be worsened by chewing or drinking sour or acidic foods. Most cases occur during the late winter or early spring.

The disease generally runs its course in about seven days. Swelling may be present on one or both sides.

Complications from mumps include epididymo-orchitis (inflammation of the testicles and their tubules), mumps meningitis, deafness, pancreatitis, arthritis, myocarditis (cardiac inflammation); and pericarditis, (inflammation of the sac around the heart), encephalitis (inflammation of the brain), oophoritis (inflammation of the ovaries) and nephritis (inflammation of the kidneys). Recent studies have suggest that the onset of juvenile diabetes is 2.3 times higher in persons who have had mumps in the previous six months, suggesting that the mumps virus may invade and damage the pancreas. (309)

Orchitis, or testicular involvement, is the complication most dreaded by young men. It seldom occurs before puberty, but may involve 20 percent or more of adults. It is usually unilateral, but occasionally involves both testicles. Pain and swelling may be severe, and varying degrees of atrophy of the testicle may ensue. Sterility, however, seldom occurs.

Long-accepted practice indicates that adequate bed rest will minimize such complications as orchitis, but definitive proof of the benefits of rest are lacking.

## TREATMENT

1. Fluid intake must be adequate to replace that lost during the fever and loss of appetite.
2. Cold or warm compresses may be applied to the neck for pain relief.
3. The diet should be simple, sugar-free, and fat-free. Spicy, irritating foods and those requiring a lot of chewing should be avoided.
4. A tepid bath or hot half bath may be given for fever.

5. For orchitis, an ice bag or cold compress to the scrotum is helpful. A charcoal compress at night may be helpful in controlling inflammation. Some have found considerable relief in the use of alternating hot and cold sitz baths as described in the section on hemorrhoids. The worst is usually over in two to four days, with subsidence of symptoms in a week or more. There is no need to consult a physician, since he can do nothing except prescribe pain-killers, which may make one sicker.

## NEONATAL JAUNDICE

Jaundice (yellowing of the skin) is the most common disorder in new-borns. It is caused by an accumulation of bilirubin in the blood. Bilirubin, a yellow pigment, comes primarily from the breakdown of hemoglobin. Enzymes break down the hemoglobin to bilirubin which then enters the blood stream. The infant's immature liver is often unable to handle the bili-rubin so it is deposited in tissues, resulting in jaundice. Bilirubin production in the newborn is two to three times greater than than in adult, because of the shorter life span of red blood cells.

Jaundice is generally not apparent until the bilirubin level reaches six to seven mg. per deciliter (dL). About 20 percent of infants have levels of 8.0 to 12.9 mg per dL, and approximately 6 percent exceed 12 mg. per dL. The jaundice is often first apparent in the upper body and progresses downward toward the toes.

In the full-term normal baby, jaundice appears about the third day and by the fifth day is disappearing. In a preterm infant jaundice may appear later, and last longer.

One type of jaundice is referred to as breast-milk jaundice. One to three percent of breast-fed infants may develop this jaundice. Peak levels of bilirubin are reached when the infant is 10 to 15 days old, and may not return to normal for as long as 12 weeks. In the past physicians frequently recommended that breast feeding be discontinued if jaundice developed, but the trend now seems to be to continue breastfeeding. Be certain to have a thyroid check on a baby who has prolonged jaundice as low thyroid function is a cause of persistent jaundice.

## TREATMENT

1. Nursing infants more frequently speeds the passage of feces which carry bilirubin out of the body. The authors of a 1982 study feel that the three to four hour feeding schedule of most hospitals actually contrib-utes to jaundice development. (297) Dr. William Gartner, professor and chairman of the department of pediatrics at the Pritzker School of Medi-cine at the University of Chicago states that feedings every two hours re-duce bilirubin levels. (298)

2. Sunlight exposure assists in the control of high levels of bilirubin. Nurseries with windows that permit the entrance of sunlight may give sufficient light exposure to prevent serious problems. (299) Infants may also be placed out-of-doors in sunlight. The eyes should be protected from direct sunlight and as much bare skin as possible exposed.

3. Many drugs taken by the mother during pregnancy, labor, delivery, and breast-feeding are felt to contribute to neonatal jaundice. Valium, sulfonamides, Orinase, hydrocortisone, Gentamicin, oral contraceptives, thiazide diuretics, and others are included in this group. (300)

4. Prematurity may also contribute to jaundice in the newborn. When labor is induced the risk of jaundice is increased. (301)

5. Charcoal is effective in lowering bilirubin levels. Activated charcoal suspended in water was given every two hours in one study done at Fort Benning, Georgia. The treatment was continued for 120 hours in normal newborns and 168 hours in premature infants, or until bilirubin levels fell. Charcoal should be begun at four hours of age to produce the maximum reduction in bilirubin levels. (302) Two to three teaspoons of charcoal per day are felt to be adequate. Stir the powdered charcoal, obtained from a pharmacy or health food store, into a little water and give with a nipple.

## OTITIS MEDIA (EARACHE)

Otitis media (inflammation of the middle ear) is a common problem in every pediatrician's office. It often follows an upper respiratory infection such as a common cold, or may be a complication of measles, scarlet fever, or other childhood disease. Males are affected more often than females, and otitis media is more common during the winter months. It seems especially prevalent among the socioeconomically disadvantaged in our society. Almost 35 percent of children have one or more attacks during the first year of life.

Children seem much more likely to develop otitis media than adults, possibly because the eustachian tubes (tubes from the back of the nose and throat to the middle ear) are wide, short and straight, lying in somewhat of a horizontal plane. This allows more nasopharyngeal secretion to enter the middle ear. The fact that babies spend so much time lying down further compromises the eustachian tube. Swallowing while lying down more readily permits nasopharyngeal materials to enter the eustachian tube. Bottle-fed babies have a higher incidence of otitis media than do breast-fed babies as mothers nursing their infants hold them in a more vertical position. Additionally, studies suggest that it is easier for a baby to suck the breast than to suck a bottle nipple. The breast yields itself to the infant's sucking, while the bottle-fed infant has to adopt a sucking technique which creates a stronger negative pressure in the eustachian tube.

Some researchers feel that allergy plays a role in the production of otitis media. An allergy may produce swelling of the eustachian tube with obstruction and retention of secretions. For this reason we recommend that children with recurrent bouts of earache be taken off cow's milk, as that is the most common cause of food allergy in children. Breast milk is the food of choice.

Symptoms of otitis media are earache, low grade fever, irritability, feeding problems, diarrhea, failure to thrive, and changes in sleep patterns. Children too young to complain of earache may tug at the ear repeatedly, sometimes beginning one to two days before the onset of acute pain.

**PREVENTION**

1. Children with recurrent ear infections should guard against forceful blowing of the nose during upper respiratory infections, as blowing may force infected secretions into the middle ear.
2. Babies should be breast-fed rather than bottle-fed. If breast-feeding is impossible, a soy-milk based formula should be used.
3. Common allergens such as cow's milk, cola and chocolate, and eggs should be avoided. Citrus fruits are another common allergen for children.
4. Drinking plenty of water will help to mobilize secretions in the throat and ears.
5. Carefully avoid using decongestants of any kind because of their vasoconstricting and drying effects.
6. Elevating the head at night will promote better drainage.
7. The patient should not smoke, or be around persons who do.
8. Avoid sugar and sweets, since they cut down on the body's ability to combat infections.

**TREATMENT**

Several studies are now showing that the use of antibiotics and antihistamines do not improve the chances of quick recovery. On the contrary, they may promote the complication of "glue ears," the filling of the middle ear with thick, tenacious secretions.

Even without treatment the course of otitis media is generally toward healing, but much can be done to make the patient more comfortable and 'encourage the body's healing mechanisms.

1. Local heat may be applied to the ear. Use a heating pad, hot water bottle wrapped in a towel, or a towel wrung from hot water. A small child may be placed on the affected side with the ear placed over the heat source. A common desk lamp held close to the ear may provide sufficient heat for relief.
2. An ice bag may be used to reduce swelling and pressure and thus decrease pain. Some patients prefer this to heat. If the ear is not draining,

one may instill a few drops of ice water into the ear as often as necessary to relieve the pain.

3. Warm glycerine or olive oil may be instilled into the ear for pain relief.

4. Steam inhalations in the form of a hot bath or shower may be helpful.

5. Hot foot baths will draw blood from the head, providing relief from congestion. Put the feet in a tub of hot water, as hot as the patient can endure. Keep it hot for 20 to 30 minutes by adding more hot water as tolerated. Keep the head cool with a cloth wrung from ice water. At the conclusion of the hot foot bath remove the feet from the foot tub and pour over them the ice water used to keep the head cool. Dress the patient warmly (particularly the feet), to prevent the slightest chilling of the skin of the extremities.

6. The diet during the attack should eliminate not only the common foods known to be allergens, but should contain no free sugars or free fats, as both decrease the activity of the white blood cells. The diet should consist of simple fruits and vegetables, with whole grain breads.

7. The ears may be treated quite effectively by a throat gargle. Use plain hot water and continue the gargle for at least ten minutes.

8. Fever treatments may be given daily. Hot baths using as hot a temperature as can be tolerated for three minutes for a child three years of age or under, and one additional minute for each year of age over. Finish off the bath with a cold water pour and a friction rub with a dry towel. Put the child to bed as quickly as possible after standing out of the hot water. Children will often sleep after this treatment.

9. A charcoal poultice may be applied to the ear. This would be particularly helpful if the ear were draining.

10. Alternating hot and cold compresses (three minutes for the hot, 30 seconds for the cold), applied to the face and sinuses will assist in decongestion of the head.

## PANCREATITIS

Pancreatitis is inflammation of the pancreas. Normal cells in the pancreas are replaced with scar tissue and calcium deposits. Mild diabetes is frequently associated with this disease. The most common causes of pancreatitis are disease of the bile ducts or gallbladder, and alcohol use. Other, less common causes of pancreatitis are injury, surgical procedures, including diagnostic procedures, electric shock, and medications, especially steroids, thiazides, azathioprine, L-asparaginase, furosemide, ethacrynic acid, phenformin, oral contraceptives, chlorothiazide, sulfonamides, tetracycline, rifampicin, estrogens, methyldopa, ACTH and valproic acid. Infectious diseases such as mumps and hepatitis may bring on the disease. Many other factors than these enter into pancreatitis; we probably do not yet know all of them. Recent studies suggest a relationship between anorexia nervosa and pancreatitis.

Symptoms include mild or severe pain in the upper abdomen. The pain may spread to the back or lower abdomen and be constant. There may be nausea and vomiting. Tenderness of the abdomen may be present. The patient may pull his legs up toward his chest and lie on his side in an attempt to relieve the pain. Food, alcohol, and vomiting may worsen the pain. There may be a low fever.

In the United States pancreatitis occurs in about 0.5 percent of the population. It is slightly more common in men than in women. Most cases will resolve with only supportive care.

After resolution of the acute phase, a certain number of patients will have recurrent symptoms at irregular intervals for months or years. This disorder is known as chronic relapsing pancreatitis.

## TREATMENT

1. Avoid all alcoholic beverages. It appears that all kinds of alcoholic beverages possess the same ability to damage the pancreas.
2. To relieve the work load of the pancreas, the patient should fast, taking only water until the symptoms subside. This is important, since food in the stomach will trigger enzyme and hormonal secretions that will stimulate the pancreas.
3. Use a low sugar diet. A high triglyceride level (caused by a diet high in refined carbohydrates) may cause pancreatitis.
4. A low calorie, low fat diet should be given after recovery from the acute symptoms. Pancreatitis is sometimes caused by high levels of fat in the blood. In the chronic form, the pancreatic enzyme lipase may be deficient, causing malabsorption of fats, making a low fat diet mandatory.
5. Adequate fluid intake is essential. Much fluid is lost inside the abdomen and it is hard to comprehend the extent of this loss because the fluid does not leave the body immediately.
6. Avoid overeating. Overeating increases stimulation to the pancreas and may cause it to overwork.
7. Medications have proven non-effective, and are often responsible for worsening the condition. Surgical procedures resulting from not infrequent misdiagnosis also result in worsening the condition. Patients may die during or after surgery
8. Caffeine, fat, and alcohol all stimulate gastric acid production and should not be used.
9. In the chronic relapsing phase, severe pain, nausea and vomiting often accompany the flareups. The patient may become habituated to painkilling drugs, making a bad situation much worse.

One of these cases, in whom the drastic procedure of total pancreatectomy was being considered, was treated conservatively by us. Frequent hot steam pack fomentations to the abdomen, charcoal taken internally and used externally as a poultice and careful attention to oral fluids and diet produced a complete remission in her symptoms.

## PELVIC INFLAMMATORY DISEASE

Pelvic inflammatory disease is an infection of the female pelvic organs. Symptoms include fever, chills, lack of appetite, nausea, generalized aching, fast heart beat, and sometimes vaginal bleeding. The patient generally has acute aching of both sides of the abdomen. Bowel movements often worsen the pain. There may be a heavy, foul smelling vaginal discharge. The pain associated with pelvic inflammatory disease may be worse on movement. It is most frequent among sexually active women in the 15 to 25 year age group. (304)

Pelvic inflammatory disease is considered to be the most frequent cause of sterility in women. About 15 percent of women have decreased fertility after a single episode of pelvic inflammatory disease. (303)

## TREATMENT

1. The patient should avoid sexual relations and douching during periods of active infection. Both may spread the infection.
2. Use a sugar-free, oil-free diet to assist the body in fighting the infection.
3. Heat may be applied to the lower back or abdomen, or hot sitz baths used for pain relief.
4. Raising the head of the bed will promote downward drainage of vaginal secretions. (308)
5. Intrauterine devices (IUDs) increase the risk of pelvic inflammatory disease. One study revealed that pelvic inflammatory disease was over four times higher in IUD users. (307)
6. Douching may induce pelvic inflammatory disease. In one study almost 90 percent of the women with pelvic inflammatory disease were vigorous douchers. The douches in patients with pelvic inflammatory disease had started earlier in life (often at age 16 or 17). It is felt that infected fluid is flushed up into the uterine cavity by the douche. (305, 306) Pelvic inflammatory disease often follows an infection of the lower genital system.
7. A hot half bath may assist the body in fighting infection. Fill a large container such as a foot tub, canner, or trash container with hot water 100 to 105 degrees. Wrap the patient in blankets to keep the body warm and have a container of ice water and washcloth for cool applications to keep the head cool. After the patient puts his feet in the water keep the water as hot as can be tolerated for 20 to 30 minutes. At the completion of the treatment lift the feet out of the hot water and pour over them the cold water used for the head compresses. Dry the feet thoroughly. The patient may rest in bed until sweating stops.
8. Hot foot baths with ice bags to the lower abdomen every four hours for

30 minutes followed by 30 minutes of bed rest increase the rate of healing, often dramatically.
9. A cold enema may be used to relieve pelvic congestion.

## PINWORMS

Infestation with the pinworm, *Enterobius vermicularis,* is worldwide
in distribution. It is the most common intestinal roundworm infestation in
the United States; from 10 to 80 percent of populations studied have had
pinworms, (249) and less than 20 percent of involved persons had any
symptoms. Pinworm infestations are generally harmless and often do not
produce symptoms. When symptoms are present, they generally consist
of itching in the anal or seat area, irritability, insomnia, and bedwetting. In
females between the ages of 18 months and 10 years pinworm infestation
is often associated with urinary tract infection. (248)

Pinworm eggs are invisible to the eye and are often carried into the
mouth on unwashed hands. The eggs may be found on table tops, bed
linen, or anything touched by the infected person. Digestive juices dissolve the eggshells and the tiny larvae are passed into the small intestine
where they grow to maturity. The females travel to the anal opening during
the night – often about two hours after the infected person goes to bed –
and deposits the eggs. When the area is scratched the tiny eggs may be
lodged under the nails or adhere to the hands to be carried elsewhere.

To check for pinworms fold a piece of scotch tape, sticky side out,
over a wooden tongue depressor or the index finger. In the morning, before bathing, press the tape firmly against the perianal regions. The tape
may be inspected for eggs using a magnifying glass or microscope. The test
should be repeated daily for six mornings. (251)

## TREATMENT

1. High doses of garlic have been reported effective. Use one to four
   cloves or four to twelve tablets daily for one week, the dosage deter-
   mined by the age of the patient.
2. A hot water enema with three teaspoons of salt to a quart of water may
   be effective. (250) Use one cup daily of this solution for a child under
   three, two cups from ages four to eight, three cups from nine to twelve,
   and one quart (four cups) from thirteen to twenty. Do not repeat the enema on the same day.
3. Wash all underclothing, bed clothes, and sheets frequently in hot water.
4. Instruct all family members to wash hands frequently, particularly after
   using the toilet and before meals.
5. Keep fingernails clipped. Scrub the nails with a brush, particularly before bedtime. Avoid nail biting.
6. Change underwear daily.
7. The infected person should sleep alone.

8. Clean sleeping quarters frequently. Even dust may become contaminated. Use ordinary household ammonia to make a solution for dampening the dustcloth.
9. Sterilize toilet seats used by infected persons.

## PRICKLY HEAT

Prickly heat is caused by obstruction of the sweat glands. Infants, overweight people, and those who live in hot, humid climates are most likely to suffer from it.

### TREATMENT

1. Avoid overheating. Use a fan or air-conditioner if one is available.
2. Wear natural, porous fabrics to encourage wicking of moisture away from the body.
3. Avoid any tight-fitting or wet clothing next to the body. Girdles and wet diapers on infants are particularly troublesome.
4. To keep the skin pores open take cool showers frequently, but avoid the use of soap.
5. Gauze, old bed sheeting, or similar material may be dipped in cool water, wrung out, and applied to the affected area as a "wet dressing." Freshen the compress every three to four minutes for an hour.
6. Drink enough water to keep the urine almost colorless.
7. Salt use should be restricted.
8. The use of ointments or oil preparations on the skin predisposes to prickly heat, as does the use of prickly heat powders.

## PROSTATITIS

Prostatitis, an inflammation of the prostate, is the most common prostate problem. Symptoms include pain on urination, and often fever. There may be a discharge from the penis.

Prostatitis is frequently treated with antibiotics despite the fact that bacteria are rarely found in the penile discharge. Antibiotics should be considered improper treatment in most cases.

### TREATMENT

1. Reducing stress may be helpful.
2. Increase fluid intake to flush the toxins.
3. Eliminate coffee, tea, alcoholic beverages, tobacco, spices, and spicy foods, chocolate, cola drinks, cocoa and nuts (particularly cashews) as these may all act as chemical irritants. Many drugs including pilocarpine, also have an irritating effect on the prostate.
4. A hot sitz bath may be taken by sitting in six to eight inches of hot water in a tub. The bath should last at least 15 minutes and be carried out

three times daily. This treatment is the mainstay of the treatment for prostatitis.

5. Avoid exposure to dampness or cold temperatures.
6. Do not sit for long periods, especially in automobiles, buses, or on train trips. Sit in a hard chair whenever possible.
7. Do not let the bladder become too full. Urinate as quickly as possible after feeling the urge. Attempt to completely empty the bladder.
8. Avoid constipation.
9. Prostatic massage is sometimes recommended, although some feel it is unwise because it may spread bacteria when they are present. The prostate should generally not be massaged during periods of acute inflammation.
10. A diet high in zinc may prove beneficial. A tablespoon or two of pumpkin seeds, which are high in zinc, may be used with each meal. Other foods high in zinc are legumes and whole grains.
11. Excessive or abnormal sexual practices may produce congestion of the prostate and supply an environment favorable for stagnation of secretion, enlargement of glands or bacterial growth.
12. Activities such as bicycle, motorcycle, or horseback riding may injure the perineum, leading to congestion of the prostate.
13. Several hours a day should be spent in out-of-doors exercise. Activity results in some degree of prostatic massage.
14. Squeezing and relaxing the muscles of the hips and perineal area will improve blood flow into the area. Work up the exercise to 50 times in each of three daily sessions.
15. Lie flat on the back, stretch the right leg over the left, and touch the floor with the right big toe. Return to the original position, and stretch the left leg over the right to touch the floor with the left big toe. Begin with as many repetitions as possible, and work up to at least 50. This exercise produces a continuous change of blood through the area.

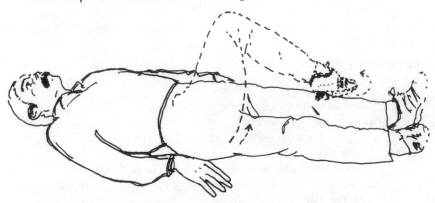

16. A short cold bath may bring relief of symptoms.
17. A hot charcoal enema promotes healing. Use one cup of hot water and one tablespoon of powdered charcoal. Insert into the rectum with a bulb syringe or an enema setup. Allow to remain as long as possible, even overnight if it can be retained.

## PSORIASIS

Psoriasis is a chronic skin condition whose cause is not yet known. The epidermis (outermost layer of skin) is produced at a rate six to nine times faster than normal, producing scales, which occur most often on the scalp, skin behind the ears, legs, arms (particularly knees and elbows), hips, and back. Itching is a frequent complaint. Skin cells normally take 26 to 28 days to develop and fall off, but in psoriasis this process may occur in four to seven days.

The disease may be mild, producing few symptoms, or it may be severe, involving most of the skin of the body. Many people with severe psoriasis suffer emotional problems, and progress to the point that they refuse to leave their homes.

There is no known cure for psoriasis, and treatment is directed toward producing and sustaining remission of symptoms.

Psoriasis is found in all age groups, but average age of onset is 20 years. It is estimated that two to four percent of the United States population suffers from psoriasis. It is one of the most common skin diseases and tends to run in families.

Stress, sunburn, any kind of trauma to the skin (pressure, scraping, excessive sun, electrical or thermal burns, etc.), fatigue, streptococcal infections and skin reactions to medication are all known to worsen psoriasis.

## TREATMENT

1. The patient should take a daily bath to assist in soaking off scales. A soft brush may be used to loosen the scales, provided care is taken not to irritate the skin, even if only slightly. White petrolatum may be applied after the bath.
2. A daily sunbath should be part of every treatment routine. Avoid sunburn as it can worsen symptoms. Several forms of artificial UV have been used, but natural light seems more helpful than an ultraviolet lamp (271). Rub white petrolatum over the skin before exposure to increase photoactivity. Some chronic forms of psoriasis are helped by a warm bath and the application of glycerin before sunbathing. (275)
3. Humidity usually has a beneficial effect on psoriasis; cold weather worsens symptoms.
4. Any measure to prevent skin dryness may be helpful. Mild cases of psoriasis may be controlled by using bath oil and applying a lubricant after the bath.

5. Emotional stress and anxiety often worsen symptoms. Daily out-of-doors exercise reduces stress.
6. If the psoriasis involves the scalp, an olive oil massage followed by a hot towel compress for 30 minutes may be used before a shampoo. Be gentle with shampooing, as too vigorous rubbing of the scalp, and particularly scratching the scalp with a mechanical device or the fingernails, can cause trauma of sufficient degree to worsen the psoriasis.
7. Several patients have reported remission of symptoms with a diet low in tryptophan. Foods containing a high level of tryptophan include milk, cheese, and meat.
8. Local heat has been helpful in some cases of psoriasis. Heat (42-46 C, 107.6-113 F) may be applied to the lesions for 30 minutes, two or three times weekly for six to ten treatments. (272)
9. A German study reports that alternating hot and cold may be helpful. Apply the heat for two minutes, cold for two seconds, (273) alternating for 15 to 20 minutes daily.
10. A diet low in sugar and free fat may produce considerable improvement.
11. White petrolatum may be applied to the troublesome areas three times a day.
12. PUVA (psoralen plus long-wave ultraviolet light) has been used for psoriasis for some years, but studies are beginning to suggest an association between PUVA and skin cancer. Other reported adverse effects of PUVA include nausea, vomiting, itching, dizziness, dry skin, headaches, skin freckling, and severe skin pain. Lupus erythematosus may worsen if present. PUVA has induced cataracts in experimental animals, and possibly in humans. (274)
13. Gentle rubbing with a pumice stone may help remove psoriasis scales in severe cases. Soaking in a tub for 10 to 15 minutes will soften the scales, making removal easier. (276)
14. Breaks in the skin are more susceptible to lesions. Avoid skin trauma.
15. A regular program of rest, exercise, and proper diet will assist the body in fighting psoriasis.
16. Avocado oil applications have been reported helpful. Others recommend a strong burdock root tea applied to the skin several times a day.
17. Some people demonstrate improvement on a gluten-free diet. Wheat, rye, barley, and oats contain gluten. (277)
18. For widespread lesions fever treatments may be used, sitting in a bathtub filled with 110 degree water. When the mouth temperature reaches 102-104 degrees the bath water temperature may be reduced five to seven degrees to maintain this body temperature for 20 to 45 minutes. Five treatments per week may be given if the patient tolerates them. Keep the head cool throughout the treatment by the use of ice bags or washcloths wrung from ice water. Three to four weeks may be

required before improvement is noted.

19. Seawater bathing has brought marked improvement in some cases of psoriasis. The program involves four to six hours of sunbathing interspersed with 20 minute intervals of bathing in the sea and the application of white petrolatum. (271) The treatment may require four to six weeks. If you don't live near the sea try adding a cup or two of sea salt to your bath water.

20. A high percentage of psoriasis patients have glucose tolerance abnormalities. (278) A health recovery diet (Appendix A) will be helpful to them.

21. A starch bath may be quite soothing. Add about one cup of starch to a small amount of slightly warm water, diluting in very hot water to form a creamy liquid which is in turn added to the bath water. Glycerin may also be added to the bath. (277)

## PYORRHEA (PERIODONTAL DISEASE)

Pyorrhea, also known as periodontal or gum disease, begins as an inflammation of the gums and extends to the ligaments and bones that hold the teeth in place. The teeth then loosen and fall out. Gum disease causes 90 percent of all tooth loss after the age of 40.

Gingivitis, characterized by redness and swelling of the gums, sometimes with bleeding, occurs before the onset of full-blown pyorrhea. The early stage is much easier to treat. Symptoms of pyorrhea are an increase in redness and swelling of the gums, bleeding, and receding gums.

A transparent film of bacteria and decomposed food particles, called plaque, is the principal cause of gum disease. If the plaque is not washed or scraped away within 24-36 hours it may harden into calculus. This calculus irritates the gums and prevents easy elimination of the bacteria from the deep recesses of the gums. Bacteria produce toxins which inflame the gums, causing them to pull away slightly from the teeth. Food particles and pus collect in the spaces, penetrate deeper, and finally attack the bone structure.

## TREATMENT

1. Emotional stress decreases the body's ability to resist gum disease. (487) Exercise neutralizes stress, and encourages healthy gums.

2. Oral contraceptives increase the risk of gum disease.

3. Do not smoke. Smokers have twice the risk of gum disease as non-smokers.

4. Use a sugar-free, fat-free diet to increase the body's ability to fight infection. A high sugar diet promotes plaque collections. In addition, laboratory animals given high sugar diets showed a decrease in bone volume. This may increase loss of the bony structures supporting the

teeth. (371) The dietary calcium to phosphorus ratio influences periodontal disease. The American diet, high in refined foods often high in phosphorus, lowers calcium levels. Calcium is important not only to the teeth, but to the bony structures which support the teeth. The fluctuations in blood calcium levels resulting from a junk food diet may play a major role in pyorrhea.

5. Brush after every eating experience and thoroughly cleanse the mouth every day. Use a soft, small toothbrush with rounded bristles and a flat brushing surface. Brush with short, horizontal strokes rather than up and down, using a wiggling motion. Hold the brush at a 45 degree angle from the teeth to allow the bristles to slip between the gums and teeth. After brushing, floss carefully. Unwaxed floss is believed best.

6. Dr. Paul Keyes of National Institute of Dental Research has developed a program which he feels will help many cases of periodontal disease. He suggests that a mixture of hydrogen peroxide and baking soda be gently massaged into the gums with a toothbrush. After a five minute wait, mix one-half teaspoon of salt in a half glass of water and rinse the mouth with it. The baking soda and peroxide kill germs and bring oxygen into the area, while the salt solution shrinks the gum tissues, giving germs less area for activity.

7. Use a diet high in fresh, raw fruits and vegetables. These foods supply vitamin C essential to healthy gums. They massage the gum tissues during the chewing process.

8. Drink adequate amounts of water. A dry mouth encourages bacterial growth. Dehydrated tissues are less able to resist infection. Saliva helps move bacteria around so they are less able to gather in colonies and form plaque. Do not breath through the mouth as this encourages dryness.

9. Warm chamomile tea may be used as a mouthwash after each brushing. It is reported as wonderfully soothing. Do not add sugar or milk to the tea. Goldenseal tea may be helpful as well. These teas possess astringent action and encourage healing.

10. The most effective remedy we have found is the twice daily use of powdered charcoal as a dentifrice. Use the brushing technique given in ____ 5. Be persistent for several months. Many have found this to be a miracle cure.

## RINGWORM

Ringworm is a term applied to fungus infections of the body, hair and nails. It is one of the most common skin infections. There are four main types of ringworm – of the scalp, trunk, nails and feet. Ringworm of the feet is also known as athlete's foot.

Ringworm of the trunk includes "jockey itch," and often begins with small, flat, red, slightly elevated ring or oval-shaped sores that may be crusted, dry, scaly or moist. The centers of the sores heal as the sores enlarge, and spread in a circular fashion. Itching, burning, or pain may be present.

This type of ringworm is spread by contact with persons having the disease, or with articles (including clothing) contaminated by them. Animals such as dogs and cats may also spread the disease.

Funguses growing under the nails result in thickened, misshapen, brittle, discolored, chalky, pitted or grooved nails. The nail is often raised off its bed. Ringworm of the nails is one of the most difficult-to-cure forms of ringworm. It may be prevented by keeping the hands dry.

Ringworm of the scalp often induces baldness which may become permanent if the fungus destroys the hair shafts. This type of ringworm is highly contagious and is most common in school children.

**TREATMENT**

1. Keeping the skin clean and dry is important in preventing ringworm. Frequent baths with thorough drying are helpful. Rub the skin and nails briskly with a coarse towel to remove the outer layer of dead skin, removing the layer in which the fungus gets its toehold.
2. People with ringworm should keep their fingernails cut short to prevent spread of the infection by scratching.
3. Infected children should sleep alone, and their linens and clothing should be washed separately from those of non-infected children.
4. Soaking the affected areas in saline solution will help remove crusts and scales. Moist compresses may be applied for 10 to 15 minutes three times a day. (280)
5. Garlic may be very effective in the treatment of ringworm. (281) The Medical Journal of Australia reports a teenage girl with ringworm of both arms who treated one arm with a prescription medication and the other with freshly cut garlic three times a day. The garlic-treated lesions healed in 10 days; the ones treated with the prescription medication took three to four weeks. Garlic may be blended in a blender with a little water and applied as a soak, compress, or poultice. *Caution:* Do not apply to raw, weepy, or ulcerated skin between toes, as injury may result.
6. Apple cider vinegar applied to the area several times a day has been reported very effective, as has castor oil, goldenseal tea, and borax.
7. For treatment of nails, pare and scrape the involved areas, and try to remove as much of the loose grainy material beneath the nails as possible. Apply vinegar with a Q-tip twice a day. Although it may require months, be persistent and often improvement will be progressive.

Too vigorous treatment of raw or weepy athlete's foot with almost any method may produce the peculiar "id reaction." This phenomenon is involvement of other parts of the body; especially the hands with an itchy or painful rash that appears very similar to the original fungus infection. It seems to be due to hypersensitivity of the body to fungus products and dead tissue, and will clear spontaneously with improvement in the original lesions.

## RUBELLA (GERMAN MEASLES)

Rubella is often called "three-day measles" and is generally a more mild form of measles than red measles (rubeola). It does have one more serious feature in that it may result in birth defects in infants born to mothers who are infected during the first three months of pregnancy. Rubella is less contagious than rubeola and many children escape the disease, entering young adulthood without immunity, and are thus able to contract the disease during pregnancy. Incubation period is from 14 to 21 days.

Epidemics often occur in the spring. One attack provides lifetime immunity. Newborns seem immune to rubella, but by the age of one year lose their immunity. (218)

Adults have relatively mild symptoms including malaise, headache, joint stiffness, and lack of energy. Mild irritation of the nose and throat membranes may be present. Lymph node enlargement may occur. The rash, which begins on the face and neck and spreads to the trunk and extremities, may be the first indication of rubella. The rash lasts about three to four days and rarely itches.

## TREATMENT

1. Use abundant fluids and a light diet free from added sugars and fats.
2. A hot half bath may be used every two hours for fever or itching.
3. Saline applications to the eyes may be soothing, as may darkening the room. (219)
4. Salt water or just plain hot water gargles may be used for sore or irritated throat.
5. Steam inhalations are useful if a cough is present.

**HOT BATHS FOR FEVERS[127]**

Keep the face and head cool. Follow all baths with 30-60 minutes reaction in bed.

| Age of Patient | 0-3 years | 4-7 years | 8-12 years | 13-19 years | 20 up |
|---|---|---|---|---|---|
| Initial Oral Temperature | 99°-103° | 99°-103° | 99°-103° | 99°-103° | 99°-103° |
| Initial Water Temperature | 106° | 106° | 106° | 106° | 106° |
| Water Temperature After 30 Seconds | 110° | 110° | 110° | 111° | 112° |
| Length of Bath | 3 min. | 7 min. | 12 min. | 13-19 min. | 20 min. |

| Age of Patient | 0-3 years | 4-7 years | 8-12 years | 13-19 years | 20 up |
|---|---|---|---|---|---|
| Initial Oral Temperature | 103° and over | 103° and over | 103° and over | 103° and over | 103° and over |
| Initial Water Temperature | 104° | 104° | 104° | 104° | 104° |
| Water Temperature After 30 Seconds | 104° | 105° | 106° | 110° | 111° |
| Length of Bath | 3 min. | 5 min. | 5 min. | 7-10 min. | 10-12 min. |

6. Isolate the patient to prevent further spread of the disease.
7. If itching is present a starch bath is often soothing. Add one cup of corn starch to about four inches of water in a bathtub. The patient may sit in the tub for 20 to 30 minutes and use a cup to dip the water onto the body parts not covered by the bath water. Pat dry to leave as much starch as possible on the skin. See item 21 under Psoriasis for method of making starch water.
8. Ice bags may be applied to swollen neck glands for 5 to 15 minutes every hour if discomfort is severe.
9. Herbal teas may be helpful: catnip tea for itching or irritability, mint tea for a stimulant if lethargic and red clover tea as a general tonic.

## SCABIES

Scabies is an infectious disease of the skin caused by *Sarcoptes scabiei.* It is also called "the itch" or the "seven year itch." Scabies is found in all social and economic groups. Contact is the sole requirement for infestation; even a handshake is sufficient. Clothing and bed linen may also be involved in transmission of the disease. Outbreaks often occur in areas where persons live in close proximity and often entire families develop infestations simultaneously.

The female mite burrows into the skin, forming tunnels in which to deposit eggs. For several weeks she will continue to burrow and deposit a few eggs a day. The eggs hatch in four to five days. Warmth, as from a warm shower or bed clothing stimulates mite activity.

The most frequent sites of involvement are the finger webs, hands, wrists, elbows, underarms, waist, and feet. In men the scrotum and penis are often involved; in women the nipples often become infected. Skin above the neck is rarely involved.

Mites are most active at night, and itching is most intense then. Scratching may induce secondary infection as well as inoculate mites in new areas. A rash may appear about a month after the primary infestation.

The disease is more common in girls than in boys, and older children and young adults are most often the victims of this affliction. Several reports have appeared in the medical literature of people who developed scabies after contact with infested dogs. (252, 253)

## TREATMENT

1. Gamma benzene hexachloride (Lindane or Kwell) has been widely used but it has been shown that this pharmacologic agent can be absorbed from the skin into the blood. Convulsions and even death have occurred in animals absorbing large amounts of Kwell through the skin. Convulsions have been reported in children after its use. (254)
2. A preparation of flowers of sulfur in a petrolatum base is a safer method

of treatment. However, it has an unpleasant odor and will stain clothing. (255) A five percent mixture may be used for children; adults may use a ten percent mixture. Sulfur ointment P.P. is 97 to 100% effective. Take a warm, soaking bath before application of the sulphur ointment. Apply ointment from the neck to the toes each night for three to five nights. Do not bathe during this period. It is best for someone other than the patient to apply the ointment as the patient may miss some areas.

3. Frequent laundering of clothing and bed linens is advised. Scabies will not survive temperatures greater than 120 F. for longer than five minutes.
4. Cool soaks, starch baths, or calamine lotion may be used for itching.
5. Garlic applications may be helpful.
6. A salve made from anise seeds is reported effective against scabies. (256)

**SHINGLES (HERPES ZOSTER)**

Shingles is an acute viral infection of nerves caused by the same virus that causes chickenpox. It has been demonstrated that children exposed to people with shingles may come down with chickenpox. (289) Stress may induce shingles. (290) Trauma, x-ray exposure, and a number of drugs have been implicated as a cause of shingles.

Symptoms of shingles are pain and fever, followed three to four days later with blister-like lesions. The skin may become red. The lesions typically are grouped over the course of a nerve or group of nerves, usually on one side of the body. The skin eruptions dry and disappear over a period of two or three weeks in uncomplicated cases, but a scar or pigmentation may remain. Pain frequently persists after the lesions have disappeared.

Shingles seems to occur most often in older people. Probably half of those who have reached 85 years of age have suffered at least one attack. Three to five persons per 1,000 may suffer from shingles.

**TREATMENT**

1. Calamine lotion may be cooling and drying. Apply the lotion generously, then cover the lesions to prevent injury. The same effect may be achieved by a solution of one-quarter cup of white vinegar to two quarts of lukewarm water applied to the crusts or blisters for ten minutes twice daily. (294) A mixture of half and half lemon juice and water or epsom salt water applied to the lesions may be helpful. The lemon water stings at the initial contact, but passes quickly. Lemon water is reported especially helpful for the itching sensation which sometimes accompanies shingles.
2. Fever treatments may considerably shorten the duration of shingles. Luella Doub, who practiced hydrotherapy for many years, recom-

mended raising the body temperature to about 102 degrees F. for 30 minutes. After a 30 minute rest period, during which the temperature returned to normal, the patient would be given a sponge bath and gentle massage. The treatment was repeated every two days until recovery.

3. Avoid chilling.
4. Heat applications may ease the pain.
5. Talcum powder or cornstarch may be soothing. (291, 292)
6. One physician reports that the application of an electric vibrator to the painful area for 20 minutes three times a day, if continued for several weeks or even months, may bring lasting relief. (293)
7. Do not open the blisters. Keep the area clean to prevent infection.
8. White petrolatum (Vaseline) may be used if the skin becomes dry and cracked as the crusts and scabs separate. (294)
9. Honey, vitamin E, and aloe vera applications have been reported to soothe singles pain.
10. A pressure dressing, such as a velcro binder, applied over the painful area may bring pain relief. (295)
11. Oatmeal baths may be quite soothing. See HOME REMEDIES for procedure.
12. Charcoal compresses may be used at night.
13. Melted paraffin applied with a cotton sponge has been reported quite beneficial during the acute phase of shingles. Apply successive layers of paraffin, waiting for each to cool and harden before the next coat. As much as one-half to three-quarters inch of paraffin may be applied in this manner.
14. An ice block massage may relieve pain after the acute phase. Rub the area for about 20 minutes with an block of ice. Pain relief may last up to 24 hours, but the treatment may be repeated two to three times per day if necessary. (296)

**TENNIS ELBOW**

Tennis elbow usually presents as tenderness and pain in the elbow and weakness of the hand. The weakness is due to discomfort when gripping objects, not to true muscle weakness.

Tennis elbow occurs more often in non-athletes than 'in athletes. Housewives, factory workers, golfers, carpenters and politicians doing a lot of handshaking are all prone to it.

**TREATMENT**

1. Rest for three to four days is essential. Rest does not mean total immobilization as immobilization leads to muscle shrinking; rest means elimination of the activities that cause pain. (493)

2. Ice may be applied for 30 to 90 minutes daily, depending on the severity of the pain. (443) Some patients find heat more soothing, particularly after the first few days.
3. Avoid cortisone injections as they may cause tendon atrophy or actually dissolve the tendon. (493)
4. Rest alone is generally not adequate to cure tennis elbow. Exercise is very important, and will help to prevent recurrences. A hand gripper may be used five to ten minutes four times a day. The elbow should be straight, and the wrist bent to stretch the extensor tendons and aid in strengthening fibrous tendons. (492)
5. Vigorously rubbing the elbow and forearm may be helpful. (494)
6. Fourteen of eighteen patients on a four to five week program of resistive exercise received complete pain relief. (495) Place the arm on a table, palm down, gripping a three pound dumbbell. Flex the wrist upward with a slight radial deviation and hold for five seconds. Return to starting position and rest three seconds. Increase the weight one pound when the exercise can be performed 15 times with ease. Continue increasing weight until eight to ten pounds can be lifted without pain. This generally requires four to six weeks of daily exercise.

    To strengthen the forearm rotators start with the arm downward and rotate the forearm 180 degrees bringing the palm upward and the dumbbell into the horizontal position. Repeat each exercise 15 times. (496)
7. An isometric exercise is reported to prevent tennis elbow. (497) Attempt a backhand swing while holding the throat of the racket with the non-playing hand. Gradually increase the strength of the pull.
8. Many players report relief by placing a band several inches wide around the forearm near the elbow and another just above the wrist. Be certain the bands are not so tight that they interfere with blood flow. (494)
9. A lighter racket with a larger grip, not too tightly strung, may help. Some aluminum or fiberglass rackets may cause less pain than wooden ones. (494) Rubbing or warming the arm just prior to playing may increase pain tolerance limits.

## TINNITUS

Tinnitus is the awareness of sound which originates in the head. Victims describe the sounds as ringing, buzzing, roaring, hissing, chirping, whistling, or whining. In some cases the sound is produced by a defective artery or vein, a clicking joint, contracting muscle, or even an insect trapped in the ear, but in many cases the origin of the sound cannot be identified.

The medical literature includes reports of sounds that could be heard by people other than the individual afflicted with tinnitus. One report tells of a child with a tinnitus that could be heard at a distance of four feet. Even dogs and cats are reported to have tinnitus which may be heard by their owners. The word "tinnitus" comes from Latin words meaning "to tinkle or ring like a bell."

A British study estimates that around one percent of the general population has tinnitus of a severe nature, but other studies suggest that nearly everyone has some degree of tinnitus at one time or another. It is frequent in people suffering with colds or sinus congestion. About 75% of deaf people report tinnitus. The frequency of tinnitus increases with age up to about the age of 70, and then declines. Some tinnitus surveys suggest that tinnitus which is heard in only one ear is 1.5 times more likely to be heard in the left ear than in the right.

A number of causes for tinnitus are known, but medical scientists are not able to prove a cause for every case. Common causes of tinnitus include severe blows to the head, drugs, otosclerosis (bone disease of the middle ear), dry, impacted ear wax, otitis, perforation of the tympanic tympanic membrane, fluid in the middle ear, epilepsy, migraine, food allergy, and a number of diseases including Meniere's disease, anemia, hypothyroidism, hypertension, migraine, and multiple sclerosis. Repeated and prolonged exposure to loud noise may induce changes in the ear which lead to tinnitus.

Through the years many types of treatment have been applied for tinnitus, but the most common treatment, and probably the most effective, is reassurance that tinnitus is a common affliction, and is not necessarily a sign of a serious problem.

Many tinnitus patients report that their tinnitus is worse when they are under stress.

Various types of surgery have been used in an attempt to cure tinnitus, but success rates are low and results unpredictable. (190) Acupuncture has been used but reported success rates are 5% or less, and some researchers feel that this degree of success may be attributed to spontaneous remission.

**TREATMENT:**

1. Avoid extremely noisy environmental situations. Occupations requiring exposure to heavy equipment, stamping operations, and power tools call for ear muffs or plugs. In the home such household equipment as food processors, blenders, vacuum cleaners may be problems. Recreational vehicles such as snowmobiles, motorcycles, highpowered boats with inadequate mufflers and such activities as shooting (especially at indoor ranges) may all induce damage to the hearing apparatus.

2. Avoid the use of alcohol. Most tinnitus patients report worsening of

their symptoms after their use of alcohol.

3. Nicotine has an unfavorable effect on the hearing mechanism and should not be used in any form.
4. Caffeine is a common cause of tinnitus and should be eliminated. Caffeine is found in coffee, tea, colas and chocolate, as well as many over-the-counter and prescription medications.
5. Marijuana and cocaine use may greatly worsen symptoms of tinnitus.
6. Many patients are being treated with tinnitus maskers, however studies are suggesting that these may be harmful. Almost all maskers available currently have the potential to produce hearing loss. (190)
7. A great number of drugs are known to cause or are suspected of causing tinnitus. Aspirin is the most commonly used of these drugs but such drugs as oral contraceptives, heavy metals used in the treatment of cancer, quinine, some diuretics, blood pressure medications, drugs used in the treatment of arthritis and thyroid conditions, certain antibiotics, steroids, anticonvulsive medications, vasodilators, drugs given to control cholesterol, folic acid, and many other drugs are causes of tinnitus. (191)
8. Fatigue may induce tinnitus. (191) A regular bed time and rising time will go far toward eliminating this cause.
9. Because stress may induce or worsen tinnitus a daily out-of-doors exercise program should be considered essential. Exercise reduces stress.
10. More and more studies suggest a relationship between allergy and tinnitus. A 1981 study listed coffee, tea, tonic water, red wine, grain-based spirits, chocolate and cheese as the most common dietary causes of tinnitus. (191) A trial period eliminating the most common food allergens (Appendix B) may be very beneficial.
11. A low salt diet may be most helpful. See the section on hypertension for simple rules for an effective low-salt diet.
12. A very low fat diet should be tried by all patients. All animal fats, and free oils, whether vegetable or animal should be eliminated. Nathan Pritikin has reported significant improvement in tinnitus on his oil-free diet. See our cookbook, SUE'S KITCHEN, for recipes and suggested menus.

## TONSILLITIS

Tonsillitis is an infection of the tonsils. The tonsils are a part of the immune defense system, functioning like the lymph nodes found throughout the body to assist in protecting the body from infection. The tonsils are located on either side of the throat, an excellent location to prevent the entrance of germs through the mouth. A Georgetown University study demonstrated that lymphocytes (white blood cells which fight infection) from the tonsils were as effective against measles as were the lymphocytes found circulating in the blood stream. Each tonsil contains 200 million lymphocytes. There are suggestions that these lymphocytes may be effective in fighting off colds, herpes, influenza, polio, and numerous other diseases. There is evidence that people who have had their tonsils removed are at a greater risk of developing some cancers than are people with intact tonsils.

Tonsillitis typically begins as a sore throat, with fever, lack of appetite, chills, headache, and muscle pain. The lymph glands in the area may become swollen. Symptoms persist for 24 to 72 hours, then gradually subside over seven to ten days. The tonsils may look red and enlarged, and pus may be seen.

For decades tonsillectomy (removal of the tonsils) has been recommended for children with repeated attacks of sore throats and colds. Physicians are now coming to understand that tonsillectomy does not decrease the incidence of these diseases. Dr. Richard A. Rapkin, medical director of Children's Hospital and professor of pediatrics at New Jersey Medical School says that cancer and airway obstruction are the only absolute indications for tonsillectomy. (282) Sixty-five children in one study were followed without tonsillectomies, and only 17 percent of them later had a similar frequency of sore throat; the balance of the study group had fewer sore throats as they matured. (283)

## TREATMENT

1. Cold applications to the throat may bring relief and shorten the attack. An ice collar or flannel wrung from ice water and changed frequently may be used. (284)
2. The patient should avoid smokers. Tonsillectomy rates have been shown to increase dramatically in children whose parents smoke. (285) As the number of cigarettes smoked increases the rate of tonsillectomies increase. (286)
3. Hot salt water gargles or throat irrigations may be soothing. Alternating hot and cold gargles will increase blood flow in the area. Goldenseal tea as an astringent gargle, with the drinking of one cup three or four times daily may be useful.

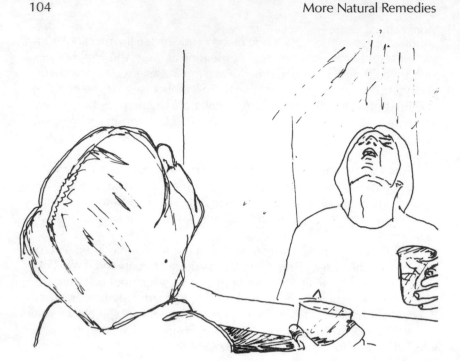

4. Adequate fluid intake is essential.
5. A heating compress may be applied to the throat between other treatments.
6. Use a simple diet, free from sugar and free fats to enable the body's immune system to function at its peak.
7. A hot foot bath combined with alternating hot and cold applications to the throat may be given two or three times a day. Apply heat for five minutes, then cold for five minutes, with three changes of each. Finish off the treatment with a cold mitten friction.

8. A charcoal tablet may be slowly dissolved in the mouth as a lozenge several times a day. It is soothing, and helps to absorb toxic products of infection and inflammation.

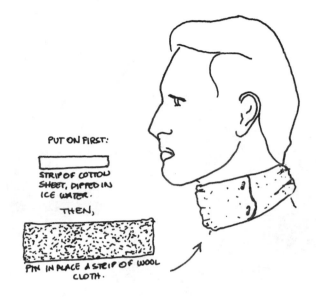

PUT ON FIRST:

STRIP OF COTTON
SHEET, DIPPED IN
ICE WATER.

THEN,

PIN IN PLACE A STRIP OF WOOL
CLOTH.

## APPENDIX A
## HEALTH RECOVERY DIET

1. Avoid all sugars including white, brown, and raw sugar, fructose, honey, syrups, jams, jellies, preserves, jello, etc.
2. Pies, cakes, sweetened desserts of any type should not be used. Make your own healthful desserts without sugar. See our cookbook for suggestions.
3. Cheese, milk and milk products are best eliminated. Milk contains leucine which has been shown to induce hypoglycemic syndrome.
4. Refined grains including white breads, crackers, saltines, white macaroni, white rice, spaghetti, and other refined grain foods should be replaced with whole grain products.
5. Extremely sweet fruits such as raisins, dates, figs, etc. are concentrated foods and are best eliminated for at least a year after beginning the diet. After a year small amounts may be introduced on a trial basis, and used if no symptoms develop. Bananas, watermelon, mangoes and sweet potatoes are all in this category. Grapes may induce symptoms in some people.
6. Caffeine, nicotine, and alcohol are all harmful to the blood sugar regulating mechanisms of the body. Coffee, tea, cola drinks, and chocolate all contain caffeine. Many over-the-counter medications contain caffeine.
7. All soft drinks contain excessive amounts of sugar or sweeteners. This includes Kool-aid. Fruit juices are concentrated foods and should be used sparingly if at all. It is much better to use the whole fruit.
8. Spices have an adverse effect on the nervous system and may aggravate symptoms. Vinegar and vinegar-containing foods may be prepared using lemon juice and salt in place of the vinegar.

## APPENDIX B
## COMMON FOOD ALLERGENS

1. Milk is the most common food allergen in the United States. Common sources of milk include whole, dried, skim, 2% and buttermilk, custards, cheese, cream and creamed foods, yogurt, sherbet, iced milk, and ice cream. Traces of milk are found in butter, breads, and many commercially prepared foods. Examine all foods for milk products such as lactose, milk solids, sodium caseinate, sodium lactate, milk fats and whey. Dr. Frederick Speer of the Speer Allergy Clinic says that all patients allergic to cow's milk are also allergic to goat's milk.
2. The kola nut family includes cola and chocolate. Both of these foods contain caffeine, as do coffee, tea, mate, cocoa and many soft drinks.
3. Corn is found in corn syrup, used in the manufacture of nearly all chewing gum, candy, prepared meats (luncheon meats, sausages, wie-

ners, bologna), many baked goods, canned fruits, and fruit juices, jams, jellies, sweetened syrups, pancake syrups and ice cream. Hominy, grits, tortillas, Fritos, burritos, tamales, and enchiladas contain corn. Cornstarch is often used as a thickener in soups and pies. Corn flour may be found in baked goods. Most American beer, bourbon, Canadian whiskey, and corn whisky all contain corn. Corn oil should be avoided. Cornmeal is used in mush, scrapple, fish sticks, pancake and waffle mixes.

4. Egg is capable of being such a potent allergen that even the odor of egg may produce symptoms. Many vaccines are egg-based. Baked goods, French toast, icings, meringue, candies, mayonnaise, salad dressings, meat loaves, breaded foods and noodles contain egg.

5. Legumes (the pea family) include peanut, soybean and licorice. Mature ("dry") peas and beans are more likely to induce reactions than are green or string beans, or green peas. Many people sensitive to the legumes are also allergic to honey, probably because in the United States honey is gathered primarily from plants in the legume family. Soybean concentrates are common in baked goods, meats, and many manufactured foods. Soybean oil is the most commonly used oil in margarines, shortenings, salad oils, etc. Peanuts are able to produce severe reactions, including shock.

6. Citrus fruits including oranges, lemon, grapefruit, tangerine and lime are common allergens.

7. Tomato and apple are common in prepared foods. Apple is found in apple vinegar, pickles, salad dressings, etc. Tomato is found in meat loaf, soups, stews, pizza, catsup, chili, salads, tomato paste and juice, and many other prepared foods. Potato, eggplant, tobacco, red and bell pepper, cayenne, paprika, pimiento and chili pepper are all in the same family as tomato.

8. Wheat and small grains such as rice, barley, oats, rye, millet and wild rice may induce allergic reactions. This group also includes brown cane sugar, molasses, bamboo shoots, and sorghum. Wheat is the most allergenic, rye the least. Rye bread contains more wheat flour than rye flour. Buckwheat is a useful substitute for wheat.
    Wheat is found in many dietary products including all baked goods, gravies, cream sauces, macaroni, noodles, spaghetti, pie crusts, cereals, pretzels, chili and breaded foods.

9. Spices and food additives often induce allergic reactions. Cinnamon is found in catsup, candies, chewing gums, cookies, cakes, chili, prepared meats, apple dishes and pies. People who react to cinnamon usually react also to bay leaf. Pepper (black and white), cumin, basil, balm, horehound, marjoram, savory, rosemary, bergamot, coriander, sage, thyme, spearmint, peppermint, and oregano often cause reactions.

Amaranth and tartrazine are possibly the artificial food colors most likely to produce symptoms. They are common in carbonated beverages, breakfast drinks such as Tang and Hi-C, bubble gum, popsicles, Kool-aid, Jello, and many medications.

10. Pork is the most common meat allergen, but oyster, clam, abalone, shrimp, crab, lobster, all true fish (such as tuna, salmon, catfish, and perch), chicken, turkey, duck, goose, pheasant, quail, beef, veal, lamb, rabbit, squirrel and venison may all induce symptoms.

## APPENDIX C
## FOODS HIGH IN PLANT STEROLS

FRUITS
Apples
Cherries
Olives
Plums

NIGHTSHADES
Eggplant
Tomatoes
Peppers
Potatoes

LEGUMES
Calabar Beans
Peanuts
Soy products

GRAINS
Cereal grains
except rye,
buckwheat, and
white rice

TUBERS
Carrots
Yams

MISCELLANEOUS
Coconut
Food yeast
Wheat germ

HERBS
Alfalfa
Anise seed
Garlic
Licorice root
Parsley
Red raspberry
Sage
Oregano

**BIBLIOGRAPHY**

1. Brunner, Lillian, R. N. and Doris Suddarth. The Lippincott Manual of Nursing Practice, 3rd Edition, Philadelphia: J. B. Lippincott, 1982 p. 242-243

2. Luckmann, Joan, R.N. and Karen Creason Sorensen, R.N. Medical Surgical Nursing; A Psychophysiologic Approach. Philadelphia: W. B. Saunders Co. 1980, p. 1030-1034

3. Human Nutrition: Applied Nutrition 36A:116-123, 1982

4. American Journal of Physiology 80:400-410, April, 1927

5. Journal of Biological Chemistry 96:593-608, 1932

6. American Journal of Diseases of Children 134:453-454. May, 1980

7. Journal of Nutrition 5:295-306, May, 1932

8. American Journal of Clinical Nutrition 6:65, 1958

9. Blood 10:35-46, 1955

10. Anatomical Records 92:33, 1945

11. Journal of Pediatrics 40:141, 1952

12. Nutrition Reviews 10:225, 1952

13. Verzar, F. International Congress on Vitamin E. 1955

14. Deutsche Medizinische Wochenschrift 109:271, 1959

15. American Journal of Obstetrics and Gynecology 71:16, 1956

16. AMA Archives of Neurology 1:312, 1959

17. Nutrition Review 20:60, 1962

18. Blood 14:103, 1959

19. Nutrition Review 20:52, 1962

20. Mitchell, et al. Nutrition in Health and Disease, 16th Edition, New York: Lippincott 1976 p. 59

21. Ibid. p. 62

22. Goodhart, Robert S. and Maurice S. Shils, Modern Nutrition in Health and Disease, 6th Edition, Philadelphia: Lea and Febiger, 1980, p. 326

23. Ibid. p. 327

24. Ibid. p. 330

25. Lancet 2:516, 1968

26. Journal of Biological Chemistry 80:431, 1928

27. Wyngaarden, James B. M.D. and Smith, Lloyd H. Jr. M.D., Cecil Textbook of Medicine, 16th Edition, Philadelphia: W. B. Saunders, 1982 p. 846

28. Ibid. p. 851

29. American Journal of Medical Sciences 107: 502-515, 1894

30. Moor, Fred, M.D. et al. Manual of Hydrotherapy and Massage, Mountain View, California; Pacific Press Publishing Association, 1964, p. 63-64

31. Landau, Barbara. Essential Human Anatomy and Physiology, Glenview, Ill: Scott, Foresman, and Company, 1976

32. Guyton, Arthur C. M.D. Function of the Human Body, Fourth Edition, Philadelphia: W. B. Saunders Co., 1974 p. 57-62
33. Silverstein, Alvin. Human Anatomy and Physiology, New York: John Wiley, 1980, p. 412-418
34. American Journal of Public Health 23:129, 1933
35. Morgan, Joe W. D.O. Cataracts and Their Treatment, Ardmore, Pa: Dorrance and Co. 1981
36. American Family Physician 24(4)111-116, October, 1981
37. Vaughn, Daniel and Taylor Asbury. General Ophthalmology, 7th Edition, Los Altos, CA: Lange Medical Publications, 1974
38. Ophthalmology 88:117-124, 1981
39. American Journal of Physiology 177:541, 1954
40. Journal of Nutrition 9:37-49, 1935
41. British Medical Journal 282:274, January 24, 1981
42. Journal of the American Medical Association 182(7)719, 1962
43. The Lancet 2:1249-50, December 5, 1981
44. International Ophthalmology Clinics 19(1) 119-225, Spring, 1979
45. Journal of Nutrition 60:157-172, 1956
46. Science News 112: August 20, 1977
47. Bellows, John G. M. D. Cataracts and Abnormalities of the Lens. New York: Grune and Stratton. 1975, p. 217
48. Cataracts. Clinical Symposia 26(3)8, 1974
49. Postgraduate Medicine, 64(5)47, November, 1978
50. Annals of Ophthalmology 11(11)1681-6, November, 1979
51. Journal of Nutrition 9:37-49, 1935
52. Proceedings of the Society for Experimental Biology and Medicine 43:85-86, 1940
53. Texas Medicine 65:48-49, January, 1969
54. Acta Societa Ophthalmologica Japonica 61:1442-1452, 1957
55. The Lancet 1:1392-1393, June 19, 1982
56. Annals of Ophthalmology 6(12)1263-5, December, 1974
57. American Journal of Ophthalmology 94(2)1263-5, August, 1982
58. The Lancet 1:472-473, February 29, 1964
59. Luckmann, op. cit. p. 1105-1112
60. Federation Proceedings 41:2797, September, 1982
61. Ibid. p. 2792
62. Ibid. p. 2801
63. British Medical Journal 1:815-819, April 14, 1956
64. Atherosclerosis 29(2)125-9, February, 1978
65. Nutrition Reviews 30:70-72, March 1972
66. The Lancet 2(7985)575-6, September 11, 1976
67. Experimental and Molecular Pathology 24:375-391, 1976
68. Experientia 30(8)910-911, August 15, 1974
69. Life and Health, March 1962, p. 5

70. American Journal of Clinical Nutrition 10:119-123, February, 1963
71. Experimentelle Pathologie 10: 1975
72. American Chemical Society Abstracts of Papers, 1982
73. Arteriosclerosis Sept-Oct. 1981
74. Nutrition Research 1(5)
75. Atherosclerosis February 1982
76. British Medical Journal May 22:1982
77. Wyngaarden, op. cit. p. 241
78. Arteriosclerosis 2:275, July-August 1982
79. Journal of the American Geriatric Society 26:284-285, 1978
80. Surgical Clinics of North America 52:359 366, April, 1972
81. American Journal of Cardiology 36(6)786-80, November 23, 1976
82. Mitchell, op. cit. p. 413-427
83. Howard, Rosanne Beatrice and Nancie Harvey Herbold. Nutrition in Clinical Care, New York: McGraw Hill Book Company, 1978 p. 318-334
84. Wyngaarden, op. cit. p. 1654-1658
85. Wyngaarden, op. cit. p. 2297-98
86. Luckmann, op. cit. p. 1977
87. Cutis 17(2)244-248, February, 1976
88. Nelson, Textbook of Pediatrics, 1979 p. 1967-1968
89. Acta Ophthalmologica 46:284-287, 1968
90. Journal of Family Practice 2(2)85-89, April, 1975
91. Wyngaarden, op. cit. p. 1627-1628
92. Life and Health, February, 1968 p. 34
93. American Journal of Nursing 81(3)519-20, March, 1981
94. Archives of Disease in Childhood 56(11)893-894, November 1981
95. The Lancet 2(8256)1150-1, November 21, 1981
96. Archives of Disease in Childhood 56(5)336-41, May, 1981
97. Pediatric Annals 6(7)68-72, July, 1977
98. Goldberg, Myron D. M.D., and Julie Rubin, The Inside Tract, New York: Beaufort Books, 1982
99. Journal of Nutrition 20:19, 1940
100. Medical Times and Long Island Medical Journal 62:313, 1934
101. Evans, Geoffry, M.D. Medical Treatment
102. Tidy, N.M. Massage and Remedial Exercise
103. Journal of the American Medical Association 230(4) October 28, 1974
104. Mitchell, op. cit. p. 359
105. Medical Press, March 7, 1956
106. Science News June 8, 1957
107. Buchman, Dian Dincin. Herbal Medicine, New York: Gramercy Publishing Company, 1979, p. 134
108. Howard, op. cit. p. 253

109. Davidson, Sir Stanley. Human Nutrition and Dietetics. New York: Churchill Livingston 1975 p. 487
110. The Medical Journal of Australia 1(5)205, March 6, 1982
111. British Medical Journal 4(5938)187-189, October 26, 1974
112. American Journal of Gastroenterology 77(9)599, 1982
113. British Medical Journal 282(6267)864, March 14, 1981
114. Bollettino Societa Italiania Biologia Sperimentale 57(23)2384-8, December 15, 1981
115. Ehrlich, David and George Wolf. The Bowel Book, New York: Schocken Books, 1981
116. The Lancet, May 12, 1962
117. Phipps, Wilma J. RN, Barbara C Long, RN and Nancy Fugate Woods RN, Medical Surgical Nursing: Concepts and Clinical Practice. St. Louis: C. V. Mosby, 1979
118. Luckmann, op. cit. p. 1891
119. Anderson, Paul. Clinical Anatomy and Physiology for Applied Health Sciences. Philadelphia: W. B. Saunders, 1976 p. 36
120. Journal of the Society of Cosmetic Chemistry 25:73, 1974
121. Journal of the Society of Cosmetic Chemistry 27:111m 1976
122. Journal of the American Medical Association 160:1397, 1956
123. Medical Letter on Drug and Therapeutics 19(15)63-64, July 29, 1977
124. RN 41:100, November 1979
125. Pageant, November, 1957
126. Wyngaarden, op. cit. p. 1993-1995
127. White, E. G. The Upward Look.
128. Proverbs 17:22 Holy Bible
129. Buchman, op. cit. p. 108
130. White, Ellen G. The Ministry of Healing, Mountain View, California, 1942
131. White, Ellen G. Counsels on Health, Mountain View, California, 1951, p. 565
132. Physician and Sportsmedicine 5:84-89, 1977
133. Physician and Sportsmedicine 6:34-37, 1978
134. Science 210:1267-1269, December 12, 1980
135. Annals of Internal Medicine 81(4)526-33, October, 1974
136. American Journal of Diseases of Childhood 136(7)652, July, 1982
137. Canadian Medical Association Journal 111(10)1048, November 16, 1974
138. Drugs 15(1)53-71, January, 1978
139. Diseases of the Nervous System 37(7)406-408, July, 1976
140. American Journal of Psychiatry 135(8)963-8, August, 1978
141. American Journal of Psychiatry 138(4)512-4, April, 1981
142. American Journal of Public Health 71(6)637-40, June, 1981

143. Abrahamson, E. M. Body, Mind and Sugar, New York: Henry Holt and Company
144. The Merck Manual, 11th Edition, Rahway, NJ:Merck and Co. Inc. 1966
145. Guyton, Arthur C. MD Function of the Human Body. Philadelphia: W. B. Saunders Co. 1974, p. 426-428
146. Landau, Barbara R. Essential Human Anatomy and Physiology, Glenview: Ill: Scott, Foresman and Co., 1976 p. 519-521
147. Silverstin, Alvin. Human Anatomy and Physiology, New York: John Wiley, 1980
148. Howard, op. cit.
149. Mitchell, op. cit.
150. Goodhart, op. cit. p. 992
151. Davidson, op. cit. p. 414
152. Ibid. p. 415
153. British Medical Journal March 7, 1964
154. Diabetes Care 5(6)634-641, November-December, 1982
155. Journal of the American Medical Association 185:102, 1963
156. The Lancet 1(8210)1-5, January 3, 1981
157. Canadian Medical Association Journal 123: 975-979, November 22, 1980
158. Diabetes Care 2(4)369-379, July-August, 1979
159. British Medical Journal 281(6240)578-580, August 30, 1980
160. Internal Medicine News 13(3)3, 41, February 1, 1980
161. Medizinische Klinik 20:337, March 16, 1924
162. Internal Medicine News, December 1, 1980 p. 5
163. Annals of Internal Medicine 82:61-63, 1975
164. Acta Medica Scandinavica 212:281-283, 1982
165. American Journal of Clinical Nutrition 29:689-690, July, 1976
166. Tohuku Journal of Experimental Medicine 130:414-412, 1980
167. Medical World News, February 19, 1965 p. 33
168. Lancet 2:716, October 3, 1981
169. Deutsche Med Wchnschr 81:514-515, April 6, 1956
170. Archives of Internal Medicine 140:707, 1980
171. Archives of Internal Medicine 140:714, 1980
172. Nursing 80 June 1980 p. 112
173. Medical Times, May 1980
174. Patient Care, April 15, 1980, p. 117
175. Brunner, op. cit. p. 646-650
176. Diabetes Care 3(1)41-43, January-February, 1980
177. British Medical Journal 284:237, January 23, 1982
178. New England Journal of Medicine 305:166, 1981
179. The American Journal of Medicine 70:201-209, January, 1981
180. New England Journal of Medicine 302(10)886-92, April 17, 1980

181. Federation Proceedings 39:1481-1486, 1980
182. Buchman, op. cit. p. 148
183. The Lancet April 11, 1964
184. Brunner, op. cit. p. 1348-1351
185. Annals of Allergy 35(4)221-9, October, 1975
186. Annals of Allergy 37(1)41-46, July, 1976
187. British Journal of Dermatology 99(3)289-92, September, 1978
188. The Lancet, 1:534, March 8, 1980
189. Science 204:506-508, 1979
190. McFadden, Dennis. Tinnitus: Facts, Theories and Treatment: Washington D. C.: National Academy Press, 1982
191. CIBA Foundation Symposium 85: Tinnitus. London: Pitman. p. 151-164
192. Weart, Edith Lucie. The Story of Your Respiratory System. New York: Coward, McCann and Geoghegan, 1964
193. Physical Therapy Review 40:368-71, May, 1960
194. Wyngaarden, op. cit. p. 369
195. Journal of Asthma Research 3(2)97-98, December, 1965
196. Brunner, op. cit. p. 207-210
197. Journal of the American Geriatric Society 18:615-22, August, 1970
198. Journal of the American Medical Association 249(6)686, February 11, 1983
199. American Journal of Obstetrics and Gynecology 135(2)279-280, September 15, 1979
200. Family Practice News, June 1, 1978
201. Journal of Sex and Marital Therapy, 5:13, 1978
202. Journal of Applied Nutrition 17(2-3)126-140, 1964
203. The Lancet 1(8181)1285-1286, June 14, 1980
204. Speer, Frederick, MD, Allergy of the Nervous System, Springfield, Ill: C. C. Thomas, 1970
205. The New York Times, October 27, 1964 "Doctors Find TV Makes Child Ill"
206. Clark, Linda. Are You Radioactive? Old Greenwich, CT: Devin-Adair, 1973
207. National Fluoridation News, October-December, 1973. Gravettey, Arkansas
208. Journal of the American Medical Association 142(16) 1286, April 22, 1950
209. Clark, Margaret. Why So Tired? New York: Duell, Sloan, and Pearce, 1962
210. Life and Health, November, 1960 p. 24-25
211. Bartley, S. Howard. Fatigue: Mechanism and Management. Springfield: Ill. C. C. Thomas, 1965
212. The Lancet 1:103, January 14, 1978

213. The Lancet 2(8103)1264, December 9, 1978
214. Family Practice News 12(12)42, June 15-30, 1982
215. Medical World News March 19, 1979. p. 11
216. Journal of the American Medical Association 241(12)1221, March 23, 1979
217. Medical World News, August 4, 1980 p. 36
218. The Merck Manual, op. cit. p. 732-734
219. Silver, Henry K. Handbook of Pediatrics, 11th Edition, p. 460-461
220. Canadian Medical Association Journal 100:626, April 5, 1969
221. Lewis, Sharon M. and Idolia Cox Collier. Medical-Surgical Nursing, McGraw-Hill, 1983 p. 1005
222. Medical Letter on Drugs and Therapeutics 18:108, December 3, 1976
223. Kordel, Lelord, Natural Folk Remedies, New York: G. P. Putnam's Sons, 1974, p. 142
224. Lewis, op. cit. p. 897-898
225. American Journal of Clinical Nutrition 34(3)428-431, March 1981
226. American Journal of Clinical Nutrition 28(11)1296-8, November, 1975
227. American Journal of Digestive Diseases 18:391-7, May 1973
228. Journal of the American Medical Association 233(10)1065-8, September 8, 1975
229. Lewis, op. cit. p. 1012-1020
230. Infectious Diseases, April, 1981 p. 16, 17
231. New England Journal of Medicine 281:1393-1396, 1969
232. Annals of Internal Medicine 80:74-76, January, 1974
233. New England Journal of Medicine 298:1-6, 1978
234. Wyngaarden, op. cit. p. 223-239
235. American Journal of Clinical Nutrition 33:561-569, August, 1980
236. Practical Cardiology 63(3)21, March, 1980
237. American Journal of Epidemiology 100:390-398, November, 1974
238. American Journal of Epidemiology 105:444-449, 1977
239. American Heart Journal 86(5)713-714, November, 1973
240. Praxis, July 1, 1948
241. Family Practice News 8(13)6, July 1, 1978
242. The Lancet 1(8160)120-121, January 19, 1980
243. Journal of the American Medical Association 173:1227, 1960
244. The American Journal of Medicine 73:348, September, 1982
245. Medical World News, August 2, 1982 p. 38
246. Medical Journal of Australia, August 23, 1980
247. Journal of Behavioral Medicine 1(1)37-43, March, 1973
248. American Journal of Diseases of Children 128:21-22, July, 1974
249. Family Practice News, April 1, 1980 p. 29

250. Rossiter, Frederick, MD. The Practical Guide to Health, Nashville: Southern Publishing Association, 1913
251. Wyngaarden, op. cit. p. 629
252. Southern Medical Journal 63(3)375, March, 1972
253. Archives of Dermatology 110:572-573, October, 1974
254. Journal of the American Medical Association 236:2846, December 20, 1976
255. Journal of the American Medical Association 236:1136, September 6, 1976
256. Meyer, George G. MD, Kenneth Blum, Ph.D., and John G. Cull, Ph.D., Folk Medicine and Herbal Healing. Springfield: Ill. C. C. Thomas, 1981, p. 241
257. Postgraduate Medicine 65(1)95-105, January, 1979
258. Brunner, op. cit. p. 821-822
259. Life and Health, Feburary 1972, p. 17,33
260. Pediatric Clinics of North America 26(2) 315-326, May, 1979
261. Wyngaarden op. cit. p. 1651
262. Medical Letter on Drugs and Therapeutics 22(16)66-68, August 8, 1980
263. Nelson, op. cit. p. 1929
264. Hoekelman, Robert. Principles of Pediatrics, p. 1394
265. Meyer, op. cit. p. 253
266. American Journal of Nursing 1299-1302, August, 1977
267. Fries, Jean MD Systemic Lupus Erythematosus: A Clinical Analysis. W. B. Saunders, 1975
268. Wynngaarden op. cit. p. 1852-857
269. Life and Health 78(2)12-13, 27, February, 1962
270. Merck Manual, op. cit. p. 732-738
271. Fitzpatrick, Thomas B. et al. Dermatology in General Medicine, 2nd Edition, New York: McGraw-Hill, 1979 p. 244
272. Archives of Dermatology 116:893-897, August 1980
273. Deutsche Medizinische Wochenschrift, December 21, 1906
274. Medical Letter on Drugs and Therapeutics 24:72-75, August 6, 1982
275. Family Practice News 2(11)15, November 1976
276. Journal of the American Academy of Dermatology 2:29, 1980
277. Sidi, Edwin MD et al. Psoriasis. Springfield, Ill: C. C. Thomas, 1968 p. 196
278. Farber, Eugene MD and Alvin J. Cox. Psoriasis. New York: Yorke Medical Books, 1977, p. 152
279. Journess Nationales de Dermatologic 103:1976
280. American Family Physician 25(1)161-3, January, 1982
281. Medical Journal of Australia 1(2)60, January 23, 1982
282. Family Practice News, October 15, 1979
283. New England Journal of Medicine 298(8)409 413, 1978

284. Journal of the American Medical Association 83:247, July 26, 1924
285. The Lancet 1:797, April 9, 1977
286. Modern Medicine, November-December, 1979 p. 42
287. Digestive Diseases and Sciences 27(3)257-264, March, 1982
288. Medical World News, December 20, 1982
289. British Medical Journal 15, January 6, 1979
290. Western Journal of Medicine 129(6)165-168, December, 1978
291. Homola, Samuel DC, Doctor Homola's Natural Health Remedies, West Nyack, NY: Parks Publishing Company 1973 p. 231
292. Modern Medicine, July 1981 p. 79
293. The Lancet 1:242, 1957
294. Epstein, Ernest, MD. Common Skin Disorders, Oradell, NJ: Medical Economics Books 1983
295. New England Journal of Medicine 306(25)1553 June 24, 1982
296. Physiotherapy 57:374, August, 1971
297. American Journal of Diseases of Childhood 136:737, 1982
298. Family Practice News 13(4)21, February 15 28, 1983
299. Pediatrics 50:131-3, 1972
300. Mothering, Summer, 1982 p. 31
301. The Lancet 1:991, May 1, 1982
302. Clinical Pediatrics 4(3)178-180, March 1965
303. New York State Journal of Medicine 80(4)635-8, March, 1980
304. Obstetrics and Gynecology 55(5)Supplement 142S-153S, May, 1980
305. Emergency Medicine, December, 1977 p. 117
306. New England Journal of Medicine 295(14)789, September 30, 1976
307. American Journal of Obstetrics and Gynecology 128(8)838-50, August 15, 1977
308. Luckmann, op. cit. p. 1891-1893
309. British Medical Journal 281:99-101, July, 1980

## INDEX